Your Life with Rheumatoid Arthritis: Tools for Managing Treatment, Side Effects and Pain

By Lene Andersen

Visit the book website at www.yourlifewithra.com

Copy editor: Holly Sawchuk   www.writerrescue.ca
Cover design: Dan Handler   www.handlerstudios.com
Author photo: Sophie Kinachtchouk   www.skphotography.ca

Published February, 2013 by Two North Books
www.twonorthbooks.com

Disclaimer:

The content of this publication is for information purposes only. Treatment of any medical condition should be developed in a dialogue between an individual and his/her physician. The information in this book is intended to assist readers in that dialogue and in making informed decisions about their health and everyday life with rheumatoid arthritis. It is not intended to be a substitute for the advice of a physician, naturopath, physical therapist, lawyer or other certified and professional service provider. While the author has endeavored to ensure that the information presented is accurate and up-to-date, they are not responsible for adverse effects or consequences sustained by any person using this book.

For my parents

Table of Contents

Foreword

I have this fantasy. In it, my RA is sitting on my green couch, perched in the middle, not making a commitment to either cushion. It looks uncomfortable, its foot vibrating with nervous tension. Its hands are clasped and tucked between its knees, shoulders hunched as it shrinks in upon itself. I am positioned in front of it, pointing at it, leveling my index finger with a determination and ferocity so intense that any minute now, a laser-bright beam will burst from my fingertip.

"You may *share* my life — I will accept that," I say in a voice that will not be denied, "but you *may not control it!*"

And the RA cowers.

I don't remember a time without rheumatoid arthritis (RA). The first symptoms of juvenile rheumatoid arthritis (JRA) appeared when I was four years old, a deep, grinding pain in my right wrist after helping my father paint the living room. Most of my childhood and adolescence was spent in and out of hospitals, fighting back flares, fighting to keep function, once fighting for my life when my JRA went systemic and attacked my heart.

When I was growing up, there were very few medications for RA and none of those available worked for me. When puberty hit, my disease went supersonic. The next four years were spent in hospitals, going home only on weekends. By the time I was fourteen, my hips had fused and I could no longer sit, so I spent my time lying in a hospital bed, waiting for custom-made hip replacements. At sixteen, I had both hips replaced, enabling me to sit again. I went home, for good this time, in a power wheelchair.

After years of hospitals, medications and doctors, I couldn't wait to be a regular teenager. All I wanted was to have as normal a life as possible and forget about having a chronic illness. So I joined my peers in high school, graduated and moved from Denmark to Canada. I got a couple of university degrees, found a job that I loved, traveled, went dancing (a lot of fun when you include a wheelchair), dated, volunteered and spent time with family and friends. In other words, I created a life. Throughout these years, my RA was on the back burner, simmered down by high doses of anti-inflammatories. It wasn't possible to forget or ignore my disease, but most of the time I managed to find ways of living well with it.

And then in 2004 the disease came roaring back, consuming everything in my life and almost killing me. I had no choice but to shift my focus and make it all about RA while I fought the battle. Thanks to a new class of drugs called the biologics, I got a miracle: for the first time in four decades of living with this disease, I responded to a medication. Although that big flare has left me more disabled and in more pain than before, I did get my life back and I'm making the most of it.

Living with RA means coexisting with an unpredictable and cantankerous shadow that will, at random intervals, try to swallow your life. Sometimes it will succeed and everything else will be derailed for a time while you and your doctor fight to get ahead. Sometimes — hopefully most of the time — life will come first while the RA mutters in the background.

Even when you find a medication that works, it doesn't solve everything. Although the RA may be suppressed, it still needs to be considered, sometimes coddled. It can be issues related to meds and their side effects or pain control and managing energy. It can be about connections with others, family and friends, developing a good relationship with your doctor or finding better or different ways to work. It can be about finding better shoes, traveling comfortably, doing chores or figuring out the least painful way to have sex. Having RA means your whole life has RA.

So how do you get to the place where it all becomes integrated in the every day, so you can focus on life, not the disease? How do you get to the "living well" part, to taking back control?

First, you need patience. It's a process, a journey of learning. Finding ways to live with and around the disease takes practice. Discovering the path to taking back control of your life means taking wrong turns and hitting dead ends. Doing it on your own can be a long and sometimes lonely road of frustration and beating your head against a wall. Having a friend along for the journey can help. Having a friend who's been there before can be even better. Someone who can show you the shortcuts and hold your hand when it gets dark and scary. A friend who'll sit with you on a comfy couch, share a bottle of wine or a pot of tea, hand you tissues when you cry and give you the skinny.

Your Life with Rheumatoid Arthritis is that friend. It's a series of books designed to be your portable go-to guide on your journey to reclaim your life. This book, *Tools for Managing Treatment, Side Effects and Pain*, is the first in a projected series of three. Each book will offer information, suggestions and tips for dealing with pretty much everything about living with RA. The goal of the series is to help you become empowered, take control of your life and go out there and live it.

Much of the information in the series and on the accompanying website (www.yourlifewithra.com) will be mined from my own experience — forty-five years of living with RA, at your service! As well, for the past four years, I've worked as Community Leader for the RA Community at www.HealthCentral.com. It's been my dream job, one that has allowed me to learn much more about the ins and outs of this disease. Together, my personal and work experience combine to create a fuller picture of everything that goes into living well with RA.

Before we get started, a couple of notes.

When you need specific medical information or advice, you should consult your rheumatologist or family doctor. I don't claim to be a medical expert and you shouldn't view me as such. There is information and suggestions in this book, but they are of a general nature. Use them to start conversations with your doctor and check with a licensed health professional before you apply them.

Not once in this book will you see the terms "RA sufferer" or "suffering from RA." There's a reason for that. There are times when living with this disease is hard. Very hard. When you start the day crying in the shower and when pain shadows your every move. On these days, it's not an exaggeration to say that you're suffering. However, I strongly believe that to identify yourself as an "RA sufferer" makes it harder to cope. How you view yourself and how you interact with the world is reflected in the language you use. If your identity is one of someone who suffers, the disease is in control, not you. Being a "sufferer" makes your life about the RA first and foremost. My goals have always been to put the disease firmly in its place and to be in charge of my life. Everything in *Your Life with Rheumatoid Arthritis* reflects that philosophy.

And lastly, about footnotes. More specifically, endnotes. Because of the annoyance factor in checking back and forth between the text and the notation, I have limited information in the endnotes to the source or links to information discussed in the text. Endnotes do not include elaboration of the discussion. The links provided in the endnotes have been checked during the last rewrite of this book in the fall of 2012 and when necessary were updated to working links.

Let's get this journey started. I look forward to sharing it with you!

Lene Andersen
Toronto, Canada
January, 2013
www.yourlifewithra.com

1
The Basics of Rheumatoid Arthritis

*"I have **what**??"*

There you are, twitching in a doctor's office and feeling slightly nauseated with anxiety, waiting to hear the news. And then they say that you have rheumatoid arthritis and your mind starts spinning with a jumble of emotions. There is the relief of finally knowing why you've been feeling like crap. Right behind the relief is shock, rolling through your brain trailing echoes of the words "rheumatoid" and "arthritis" like a passing thunderstorm and... Hang on. Isn't that what old people get? And what does *chronic* imply? Does this mean your life is over?

Before we go any further, take a deep breath. It will help with the dizziness.

RA — as it is known among those of us who live with it — is a chronic illness, and that means you'll have it for the rest of your life. I'm not going to lie to you. It's not always a dance on fragrant pink rose petals. In fact, it can sometimes be a downright dance on thorns. You will have challenges that you never imagined would be part of your life, and there are times when you will be decidedly unhappy. In the end, you will be the stronger for it. Much of the time, it isn't going to be all about the illness. Sure, you will share the rest of your life with a partner you can't get rid of, but there is no reason why you shouldn't have a career, relationships, children, friends, laughter and all the other things that are part of life.

One of the keys to living well with RA is to find a way to take back control of your life. The more you know about your new companion, the more in control you'll feel. Keep educating yourself, even when it makes you anxious. To prevent your anxiety from leading straight into a hyperventilating panic attack, make sure you choose sources of information that are responsible and reputable. Examples include The Johns Hopkins Arthritis Centre (www.hopkins-arthritis.org), About.com's site on rheumatoid arthritis and joint conditions (arthritis.about.com) and HealthCentral's RA community (www.healthcentral.com/rheumatoid-arthritis).

In the interest of full disclosure, I should mention again that I've worked for HealthCentral since 2008. I don't say it's a good website just because I work there — we provide solid, up-to-date information from a positive point of view. So do many other sites and you will soon find your favorite.

The silver lining — and yes, there is one — is that if you have to have RA, now is a pretty good time for it to happen. There are incredible new treatments available that make it possible for more people with RA to live close to normal lives than ever before.

This book focuses on helping you learn how to manage your RA so you can get on with your life. Part I of the book will give you more details about the different treatments for RA and where they can lead you. It's an unfortunate reality that all medications may have side effects, but many of them can be managed. Part II of the book has information on how to manage mild to moderate side effects, with tips that can help make your experience with the meds a positive one. Another aspect of managing your RA is finding ways of coping with the pain that is often part and parcel of this condition. Part III has suggestions for your pain management toolbox.

Before we dive into the nitty-gritty of meds, side effects and pain control, a short introduction to RA is in order. You've probably already found information about the disease, but bear with me. This chapter frames the discussion in the rest of the book. So with no further ado, I'd like to introduce you to RA.

What is RA?

Rheumatoid arthritis is not the kind of arthritis you get as you age. That's osteoarthritis, also known as "wear and tear arthritis," which can happen as you grow older or after an injury. RA, on the other hand, is a chronic autoimmune disease that causes inflammation, primarily in the joints. However, RA can also cause inflammation in tendons and internal organs. RA is called a systemic disease because it affects different parts or systems of the body.

RA is part of a family of conditions called autoimmune diseases that also include multiple sclerosis, lupus, juvenile arthritis, schleroderma and many more. When you have an autoimmune disease, it means that your immune system gets confused and attacks your body. Instead of protecting you, your immune system undermines your health. In RA, this attack causes a chronic inflammation in the synovial tissue that surrounds your joints, as well as in similar kinds of tissue lining certain organs. In your joints, this inflammation eats away cartilage, which provides a cushion between two joint surfaces, and destroys tendons and bones. When this kind of damage happens, the joint may become deformed and lose function. Chronic pain may be a big part of having RA and is caused by inflammation and, for some, damage to the joints.

At this time, there is no cure for RA, but it can be treated. Recent advances in medication mean it is now much more possible to achieve remission, stopping the progression of the disease and preventing damage to your joints and other parts of your body. And that means you have a better chance to continue living your life.

What Causes RA?

The cause of RA is still unknown, but research is continuing in this field. At this time, indications are that a mix of genetic and environmental factors can start the immune response leading to RA in people who are predisposed to the disease.[1] Many environmental factors have been suggested as being involved in triggering RA, including various kinds of infections, bacteria or fungi. There are clues to this connection in studies of people with RA, as well as mouse models of arthritis, but so far no connection has been proven, and this is still a subject of intense investigation.[2]

At present, the strongest environmental connection to RA is smoking, through some as yet unknown interaction with genetic predisposition. Keep in mind that many more people smoke than develop RA and that some people who have RA have never smoked, so there is more going on in this process. Still, quitting smoking is always a good idea — if nothing else, your lungs will thank you for it.

Another piece of the puzzle deals with the predisposition to the disease. RA has a genetic component, which means it can run in families. If this makes you hesitate about starting a family or worry about the kids you already have, be assured that it's far from certain that you will pass it on to your children. First-degree relatives — that is, siblings or children — of a person with RA only have a 5% risk of developing the disease.[3] This means they have a 95% chance of *not* getting RA.

Research is beginning to show us part of the larger picture, but there is still much we don't know about this disease and its cause. What is known is this: an unknown trigger combines with a genetic predisposition to develop an overactive immune system that creates inflammation in the joints and other systems in the body. That sounds very general and vague, but it's a place to start. All over the world, dedicated researchers are chasing the answers. One of these days, they'll have the breakthrough.

Who Gets RA?

One in one hundred people develop RA, approximately 1% of the population in any country. RA can start at any age, including during childhood, but most commonly happens between the ages of twenty-five and fifty.

Many autoimmune diseases are more prevalent in women than in men and this is also the case for RA. It affects women three times more often than men.[4] Many women who have RA report a flare of their symptoms in the days before their periods start — as if regular PMS wasn't enough! As well, 65% of pregnant women with RA will go into remission, although the RA frequently comes back about six to eight weeks after the baby is born.[5] Both of these factors seem to indicate a possible hormonal connection to RA, although the specifics of this connection are still unknown.

How is RA Diagnosed?

The quest for a diagnosis starts when you visit your family doctor to talk about pain and swelling in your joints, fatigue and morning stiffness. Your doctor may send you for blood tests and hopefully refer you to a rheumatologist. If they don't, request a referral. When you have RA, the earlier you get diagnosed and start treatment, the better your chances for a good outcome.

A diagnosis of RA should be made on the basis of taking a medical history and a physical exam, with blood tests used as possible confirmation. A good rheumatologist will be able to make a diagnosis of possible or definite RA even without blood tests.[6]

There are two blood tests that your doctor can use to help diagnose RA. They are Rheumatoid Factor antibody (RF) and the anti-cyclic citrullinated peptide antibody (anti-CCP or ACPA).

Most family doctors will test for RF. If it is positive, they may tell you that they suspect RA and refer you to a rheumatologist. A positive Rheumatoid Factor is not a sure-fire indication that you have RA. This test can also be positive in about 5% of healthy individuals, people with other types of rheumatic diseases and people with infections.[7]

The anti-CCP is a newer blood test that appears to be more reliable for confirming a diagnosis. Until now, the antibody has been found almost exclusively in people who have RA and in people with very few other conditions. As well, this test can be positive up to fifteen years prior to developing RA. Therefore, the anti-CCP can be an important tool in identifying who will get RA before other signs of the disease are present, making it easier to protect joints from damage. Rheumatologists believe this early identification, combined with promising drug research, may in the future make it possible to turn off this disease before it starts.[8]

One or both tests — RF and anti-CCP — is positive in most people who have been diagnosed with RA. When these tests are positive, you have seropositive RA. Approximately 20–30% of people who live with RA are seronegative, which means their blood work does not show a positive RF. Most family doctors are not aware of the intricacies of RA, and therefore may not refer you to a rheumatologist if your blood work is negative. If that happens, find a couple of articles about seronegative RA on a reputable website, show them to your doctor and ask for a referral.

When you see a rheumatologist, they may order x-rays to check for joint damage. Inflammation can cause damage for some time before it is visible on x-rays, so if your images are normal, it doesn't rule out RA. In fact, studies have shown that damage can be visible on an MRI up to six months before it is seen on an x-ray.[9] So, if your doctor rules out RA based on no visible damage on your x-ray, consider asking for an MRI. It can be useful both in diagnosis and in following the possible progression of inflammation and damage in your joints.

Unfortunately, there is no one test that can say "you have RA." A doctor will make a diagnosis based on your report of joint pain, morning stiffness and fatigue and finding swollen joints when they do a physical exam. Blood tests and x-rays are used to confirm the diagnosis, not as primary diagnostic tests. Your doctor may also order other tests to check for conditions that can mimic RA, such as lupus, Lyme disease and others.

If your family doctor or the rheumatologist to whom you were referred dismisses the possibility of RA, push for a second opinion. It is an unfortunate reality that it sometimes takes more than one doctor before a diagnosis is made and treatment can begin.

What About the New Criteria?

You may have heard about new criteria to diagnose RA. There have been many misunderstandings about these criteria in the media, even the medical media. Here is a brief clarification.

In August of 2010, an international working group of rheumatologists from The American College of Rheumatology and The European League Against Rheumatism (ACR/EULAR) released a new set of classification criteria for RA. The biologic medications "are the driving force behind this change. It is because of the revolutionary impact of these types of drugs that the goal of treatment is now 'to prevent individuals from reaching the chronic, erosive disease state that exemplifies the 1987 criteria for RA.'"[10] The new criteria are intended to be used in clinical studies to identify people at an earlier stage of RA. This way the studies can look at how effective treatments are in preventing damage and disability over time.

Some doctors are adapting these criteria to use as tools to diagnose RA. The working group cautions that this can only be a limited application as "clinicians may be able to diagnose an individual who has not met the classification criteria definition or who has features that are not a component of the classification criteria."[11] In other words, you may have RA even though you don't meet the new criteria. Although the criteria may help doctors identify some cases of early RA, further testing is needed to assess how effective they can be as a diagnostic tool.

What is a Flare?

When your RA flares, it means that the disease has becomes more active, making your joints swell and your pain and fatigue increase. It feels sort of like you're wearing a damp, lead-lined comforter at all times, making you use more energy to move, which makes you much more tired.

When you're flaring, it is very important to contact your doctor as soon as possible so you can find a medication to beat the flare back into submission. The sooner you get treatment to suppress your RA, the better your joints are protected from damage and the sooner you can get back to your life. The treatments that are available to help control your RA are the focus of Part I of this book.

Predicting the Unpredictable

One of the toughest aspects of living with RA is the unpredictability of it all. Your symptoms can come and go with seemingly no rhyme or reason, and it can make it very difficult to regain a sense of control. Keeping a symptom diary can help you get an overview of how RA affects your life and how your life affects your RA.

You can approach this the old-fashioned way, by buying a notebook at an office supply store, or the fancy way, by setting up a spreadsheet on your computer. Create several headings for things to track each day. Your headings could include the following:

- Symptoms (such as swelling, stiffness, fatigue and pain)
- Activities (at work, at home and recreation)
- Food (list what you ate for each meal)
- Weather (including temperature, humidity, changes from sunny to raining and vice versa)
- Emotional well-being (such as good and bad moods, when you're feeling stressed, etc.)

Fill in these fields every day for three to four weeks — this is long enough to help you identify patterns, but not so long that the process starts to drive you crazy. Then sit down and take a look at your symptom diary. Was there something going on in your life in the time leading up to a flare? Do particular symptoms seem to be related to when you take your medication, so might they be side effects? Did the weather turn? Did you eat specific foods before your symptoms got worse? Do any of your activities seem to trigger flares more than others?

A symptom diary gives you the ability to take a step back and look at the bigger picture, which can help you discover triggers to flares and patterns with side effects. This can help you modify the way you go through your day or find help for a particular side effect, giving you more control over your experience with RA. A symptom diary can also be a valuable tool for your doctor. Showing evidence of patterns to your rheumatologist can help you and your medical team address problems, which improves your care.

If you have a smartphone, you can download an app that will do all this for you. Apps that track your symptoms and how they interact with what you do are particularly prevalent on the iPhone and iPad platforms, although you can also find some for Android phones. In the fall of 2012, the Arthritis Foundation released Track + React, developed specifically for people who live with one of the one hundred different kinds of arthritis. It is available for iPhone, iPad and Android and you can download it at www.arthritistoday.org/tools/track-and-react/track-and-react-app.php. WebMD's Pain Coach is aimed at people who live with chronic pain from a number of different conditions. It is available for iPhone and iPad and can be downloaded at www.webmd.com/webmdpaincoachapp. Both of these apps allow you to graph the relationship between what you do and how you feel, as well as create reports that you can share with your doctor. Both apps are free.

RA is a complicated disease and there is an overwhelming amount of information about it available online and in text books and scholarly journals. This chapter was meant as a brief overview to serve as a foundation for the discussion in the rest of the book. If you're interested in more detailed information, the Internet is a good place to start, as long as you stick to reputable websites.

And now for the meat of the book. Next up: treating RA.

PART I:
MEDICATIONS FOR
TREATING RA

2
Medications Introduction

When I was growing up, the treatments used to control rheumatoid arthritis were limited to steroids and injections of gold salts. That was ionic chemical compounds of gold — yes, that gold — injected in my rear and no, my arse didn't suddenly increase in value after the shots. By the time we entered the new millennium, a number of other medications had been added to the list and a quantum leap in RA treatment was underway.

This part of the book deals with issues surrounding medication for RA. It includes chapters on the rationale for taking medication, the kinds of meds that are available to treat the disease at the time of writing this book, financial assistance programs, remission and opioids and treatment agreements. They are intended to get you started on the journey of researching and understanding the treatment your doctor suggests. More detailed and up-to-date information on the individual medications — and the meds developed between the time of writing and when you read this book — is available from your doctor, the library and your best friend, the Internet.

Researching Medications

On the Internet, start with the manufacturer's page about the medication you're researching, but remember their job is to sell the drug. That means that although they must have a page with information on possible side effects, the website will likely err on the side of rosy. Branch out, hit RA websites, Wikipedia and sites with detailed information about medications such as drugs.com and about.com.

There are two general groups of medications used to treat RA: drugs that are aimed at controlling the illness and drugs used to treat the symptoms.

Disease-modifying antirheumatic drugs (DMARDs) and the biologics are used singly or in combination to control inflammation, with the goal of suppressing active RA and inducing remission (see Chapter 8).

The second group of medications is composed of nonsteroidal anti-inflammatory drugs (NSAIDs), steroids and other types of painkillers. The meds in this group are used to relieve symptoms of inflammation and pain, but do not suppress RA. It's quite common to use both DMARDs and painkillers together to manage RA.

In your research, you'll come across many mentions of side effects. Usually, these are fairly manageable, although as with all other types of meds, there is a possibility of rare, serious side effects. Part II of this book will explore ways of managing different kinds of side effects in more detail. But first, let's take a look at the meds.

One note before you continue. This topic can be a bit dry and overwhelming. I've done my best to present the information in something close to English, rather than medical jargon. If you run up against something you don't understand, ask your doctor or check Google and online RA communities.

3
Why Take Medication for Your RA

"I don't want to take toxic medication."

Close on the heels of getting a diagnosis of RA comes the conversation about medication. Your rheumatologist will assume you want a prescription, but for many, this is a moment when they (metaphorically) make like a dog and dig all four paws into the ground, fighting the idea. Usually while quoting a variation of the notion of medications being toxic.

If you've been diagnosed with a chronic illness, it's important to stay healthy, right? That means eating a balanced diet of healthy (preferably organic) foods, getting exercise and being careful to put only good things in your body, right? And that means no chemicals, right? So no medication, especially the scary ones that come with words like "chemotherapy drug," "immunosuppressant" and "potentially serious side effects."

Well, yes and no. It is indeed important to stay as healthy as you can and to take good care of your body. Now that you have RA, taking good care of your body also means taking medication.

The Three Ds and the Mortality Gap

At this time, there is no cure for RA.

RA is a chronic illness. You will have it for the rest of your life.

The reality of what it means to be diagnosed with RA is not a pleasant thing to face. The words can ring in your mind for days, weeks or longer and it's normal to want to stick your head in the sand and pretend it isn't happening. But it is necessary to look at what scares you the most. To make good choices, you need all the information, and the fact that the meds sound scary is not the full story.

RA has consequences that I call the three Ds. Left untreated, RA will *damage* your joints, which can cause *deformities* that change the appearance of your body. Such deformities can include various degrees of contractures — i.e., being unable to fully stretch or bend the joint — leading to restricted mobility and disability. When I was diagnosed with RA, there were no effective treatments. Because of this, my RA caused so much damage, deformity and *disability* that I had to start using a power wheelchair at the age of sixteen.

And while I'm at it with the scary talk, there's also the mortality gap. Statistically, people with RA die sooner than others. When you have RA, you have a higher risk of comorbidities. This means other illnesses and conditions existing side by side with RA, such as hypertension (high blood pressure), heart disease and diabetes. The type of systemic inflammation and problems with the immune system that happen in RA seem to increase the risk of comorbidities and result in poorer outcomes. As well, people living with RA may not receive the kind of preventive care necessary to good health. My guess is that this is because RA and its treatments take up so much room that health maintenance can fall by the wayside.[12]

Does that mean we're doomed? Not necessarily. If you're feeling panicked, take a deep breath — paper bags are good for this purpose — and read on.

A Shift in Perspective

We grow up learning that medication should be used only when you absolutely need it. That you should let your body heal naturally whenever possible and that the chemicals in medication aren't good for you when taken for too long. The thinking of a healthy person is often that *medication is bad*. When you have RA, you need to change gears and switch your perspective to *medication is your friend*. And yes, that includes a drug called methotrexate, even though it's a particularly interesting shade of yellow with lime green overtones.

Medication protects you. The goal of treatment is to suppress your RA. This means the disease won't be busy eating the cartilage in your joints and they will be protected from damage. If your joints are protected from damage, you will not get deformities and without deformities, you will be protected against disability. Medication protects more than your joints, also affecting the systemic impact of the disease, improving, among other things, your heart health. Taking medication protects your ability to continue living your life as fully as you can. It allows you to buy your own groceries, continue to work, parent your children, be there for your family, walk the dog, cook dinner and all the other little things that make up your life.

Revolutions in Treatment

It used to be that there was a small handful of medications to combat RA. If none of them worked well, you picked the one that worked the best and kept your fingers crossed. For most, the prognosis was poor. Sooner or later, you would travel the road of the three Ds, damage and deformities gradually making it difficult to move and causing high levels of pain. You would lose your ability to walk, need surgeries such as joint replacements and even then, some level of disability was almost inevitable.

Then came methotrexate.

Originally a chemotherapy drug used for cancer, methotrexate was approved for use in rheumatoid arthritis in the late 1980s. This is usually the point when people start looking really worried — chemotherapy drug? For RA?? Don't fret. When used for RA, methotrexate is given in much smaller doses compared to when it is used for cancer, and side effects are much less than the drastic ones often associated with chemotherapy. More importantly, methotrexate was the first step in the treatment revolution, helping people with RA go into remission rather than just slow down the progression of the disease.[13]

Methotrexate is still around — in fact, it is currently considered the "gold standard" of RA treatment. This means that it is usually the first drug to be prescribed, especially in moderate to severe cases.

23

And then came the biologics.

In the early 1990s, I went to a lecture given by Dr. Edward Keystone, a prominent Canadian rheumatologist. He described RA treatment of the day as a sort of unilateral carpet-bombing of the immune system, destroying everything in sight. He went on to say that researchers were looking for a weapon that could target specific cells and leave the rest of the immune system intact. The biologics are this weapon.

Enbrel was the first biologic medication. It started changing people's lives around 1998 and now, fourteen years later, there are nine biologic medications on the market. A biologic medication "copies the effects of substances naturally made by your body's immune system. "[14] They are genetically engineered to interfere with "biologic substances that cause or worsen inflammation. "[15]

For many, these medications are miracles in a syringe or IV bag. They enable many more people with RA to function at a level previously unheard of. In fact, these medications have had such a profound impact on RA that we still don't know how far it's possible to go. The prognosis — a doctor's assessment of how the illness will progress — has changed drastically. Because there are now very meaningful options for treatment, the approach to treating RA is also changing. People with RA are increasingly treated early and aggressively, and this often means that joints are protected before the damage starts. It means living normal lives, it means less surgery and the possibility of not seeing deformity and disability for decades, possibly ever. More detail about biologics is included in Chapter 4.

The biologics don't just improve your RA prognosis, they also seem to improve your general health, as well. My doctor ordered a series of blood tests after I'd been on Humira for about a year and I saw the miracle for myself. I'd been severely anemic since I got RA as a child over forty years ago. Now I wasn't. In fact, my doctor told me that if she only looked at my blood tests, I would look like a normal, healthy woman. That day, I cried in my doctor's office and they were tears of joy.

And I'm not the only one. Studies have shown that these types of medications can cut the risk of cardiac incidents in half and improve outcomes if they do occur. Inflammation plays a role in the health of your heart, and when you suppress the inflammation, you suppress the risk of cardiac events. In addition to reducing rates of heart attack and stroke, biologics can substantially reduce rates of infection and cancer.[16] That means narrowing the mortality gap and increasing the average life span of a person with RA.

Considering the pros and cons of taking any medication is an important part of the decision-making process. Although some do not respond well to medication, most people do pretty well with very manageable side effects (see Part II: Managing Side Effects). That said, you can't close your eyes to the possibility of developing more serious side effects (see Chapter 27). As you make your decisions about medication, remember to keep it all in perspective — the risk of serious side effects can be significantly lower than the risk of getting into a serious car accident, and most of us get in a car every day without thinking about it. You have to weigh the risk against the possible, even likely, significant benefits. At the end of the day, it comes down to realizing that you cannot control RA with the powers of your mind. Given that unfortunate fact, what is your life worth? If there's a possibility of reducing the pain, fatigue and hardship of active RA, of getting back to your life with your disease pushed to the background, what would your answer be?

4
Medications to Suppress Your RA

"Do the meds come with a pronunciation guide?"

The first stop on our tour of the different drugs used to treat RA is a visit to the meds designed to control the illness. These kinds of medications get right to the root of the problem, modifying the disease or targeting an immune response. When your rheumatologist hands you a prescription for this kind of medication, it is in the hope that it will suppress your RA, thereby protecting your joints. This will prevent the three Ds described in Chapter 3 — damage, deformities and disability — as well as improve your general health. The goal of treatment is to help you go into remission (see Chapter 8).

DMARDs

DMARDs (disease-modifying antirheumatic drugs) are medications that are intended to do exactly what the name implies: modify your disease. When they work, they suppress disease activity, which reduces the inflammation in your joints. No inflammation means no damage. When they work well you have a remission, which means there is no evidence of disease activity in your body. Usually, you have to continue taking the meds to stay in remission. For most people, stopping the medication will cause the RA to come back.

DMARDs is a large, general category of drugs that include medications specifically developed for RA as well as meds originally used for other diseases, but which were found to be effective for RA. DMARDs suppress many parts of your immune system. You may remember from the overview in Chapter 1 that RA is an autoimmune disease in which the immune system attacks itself. These medications inhibit or stop that response.

Methotrexate has been considered the first-line treatment for RA since the early 1990s.[17] Methotrexate is a chemotherapy drug. I can hear you starting to get anxious, but relax, it's not as bad as all that. When treating RA, methotrexate is used in much smaller doses than as chemotherapy for cancer and usually has completely manageable side effects. It works by suppressing your immune system, making your RA symptoms subside. Since your immune system is suppressed, you may also be more vulnerable to developing infections. Chapter 17 will discuss how you can manage the risk of infections.

Another type of DMARD is Plaquenil, also know by its generic name hydroxychloroquine, which was originally a malaria drug, but can be effective in managing RA. Other medications in the DMARDs category include Arava (leflunomide) and Azulfidine (sulfasalazine). In Canada, the UK and many other countries, the brand name for sulfasalazine is Salazopyrin.

The new forms of immunosuppressants include the biologics, which work by targeting specific parts of your immune system.

Biologics

Around the year 2000, a massive revolution happened in RA treatment. Like many events of radical change, it brought with it the promise of freedom and independence. Contrary to the usual revolutionary trend, these promises were actually kept, giving people living with RA a better chance at normal lives than any previous treatment had offered. The biologic class of drugs changed the prognosis so completely that at the time I write this, we don't know how far it's possible to go. What we do know is that the biologics mean we are no longer doomed to a gradual progression of damage, deformity and disability.

This type of medication targets "molecules on cells of the immune system, joints, and the products that are secreted in the joints, all of which can cause inflammation and/or destruction."[18]

There are several kinds of biologics:

27

- **TNF blockers or TNF alpha inhibitors**
  The tumor necrosis factor (TNF) is an "immune cell protein that kills cells that appear abnormal and stimulates autoimmune reactions like inflammation."[19] TNF blockers include Enbrel (etanercept, the first biologic, introduced in 1998), Humira (adalimumab), Remicade (infliximab), Simponi (golimumab) and Cimzia (certolizumab pegol).

- **Interleukin-1 inhibitors**
  Interleukin-1 is another type of inflammatory substance and is inhibited by the biologic Kineret (anakinra). This drug is rarely used for RA, as it tends not to work effectively.[20]

- **Interleukin-6 inhibitors**
  Actemra (tocilizumab) is a medication designed to inhibit the inflammatory substance called interleukin-6.

- **T-cell costimulation inhibitors**
  T-cells are another mechanism involved in inflammation — aren't we lucky there are so many options for creating inflammation? — and can be inhibited by the drug Orencia (abatacept)

- **B-cell depleting drugs**
  B-cells are activated in cases of inflammation, such as RA. The medication Rituxan (rituximab) depletes B-cells, but tends to be held in reserve for people who do not respond to TNF blockers.

JAK Inhibitors

In November 2012, a new type of medication was approved by the FDA. Xeljanz (tofacitinib) is a Janus kinase (JAK) inhibitor. Whereas the biologics work to inhibit proinflammatory cytokines from outside the cell, JAK inhibitors work on a different inflammation pathway. They are small molecule drugs that fight inflammation from within the cell, inhibiting the JAK pathway.[21] Xeljanz is a tablet, not an injection or infusion. More JAK inhibitors are in development.

The medications listed above are those that are available at the time of writing this book. More biologics and JAK inhibitors are coming down the pipe, giving all of us who live with this illness more reasons to hope than I have seen in my over forty years of living with RA. In only fifteen years, we have gone from carpet-bombing the immune system to treatments that target specific immune responses. From my perspective, this is nothing short of a miracle.

The biologics are what I call The Big Drugs. They are designed to help people who do not respond to medications such as methotrexate and Plaquenil. When you're in that situation, you have a big problem that needs a big solution. And when you have a big solution, it usually carries a larger risk than other types of medication. The biologics do come with an "interesting" number of possible side effects, some of which can be quite serious. The reasons involved in the decision to switch to the biologics were covered in more detail in Chapter 3, and more information about what to do about side effects can be found in Part II of the book, Managing Side Effects.

5
Medications to Manage Pain

"Pain be gone!"

The second stop on our tour of medications for RA is drugs that are intended to give you symptomatic relief. That means they do not address the underlying cause (RA), but give you relief of symptoms like inflammation and pain. These types of medications can be an important tool to help you function and get through your day.

Nsaids

The term NSAIDs is short for nonsteroidal anti-inflammatory drugs. These are medications that reduce inflammation but are not steroids. Although there are many painkillers on the market, the ones primarily used to treat the symptoms of pain and inflammation that come with RA are two kinds of anti-inflammatory drugs.

Before I move on to discussing anti-inflammatories, it's necessary to talk about what causes inflammation. The cells in our bodies produce a family of chemicals called prostaglandins. These chemicals have a number of important functions, including promoting and inhibiting inflammation, fever and pain. They are "part of a complex regulatory network that modulates the actions of immune cells and the surrounding microenvironment."[22] I'm sure you and I would argue that promoting inflammation is not a terribly important function. However, in addition to their regulatory duties, prostaglandins also support blood clotting and protect the stomach lining from the damage that could be caused by acid, so they're kind of necessary.

Within the cells, there are two types of cyclooxygenase enzymes that produce prostaglandins: COX-1 (responsible for protecting the stomach) and COX-2 (primarily present at places where there's inflammation).[23] NSAIDs work by blocking these enzymes, thereby reducing prostaglandins and in turn reducing inflammation, fever and pain.[24]

NSAIDs have been around for a long time and there are a large number to choose from. Most of the available NSAIDs are "nonselective" — that is, they inhibit both COX-1 and COX-2.

Aspirin, or acetylsalicylic acid (ASA), has been around since the mid-1800s and is a traditional workhorse for pain.[25] Aspirin is also used to prevent heart attack and stroke and in such cases is taken in small daily doses on the advice of a doctor. When used for RA, aspirin needs to be taken more frequently (usually four times a day) and is therefore often farther down on the list of recommendations for pain management.

Other over-the-counter NSAIDs include Advil (ibuprofen) and Aleve (naproxen, also available in prescription form). Prescription NSAIDs include Mobic (meloxicam), Relafen (nabumetone), Voltaren (diclofenac), Orudis (ketoprofen) and numerous others.

Topical anti-inflammatories like Pennsaid are a relatively new addition to this group. You place a few drops of liquid on the place it hurts — for instance, a knee or an elbow — and rub it into the skin.

Another type of NSAIDs is called COX-2 inhibitors. Traditional NSAIDs can be very hard on the stomach, potentially causing bleeding ulcers and other stomach distress. COX-2 inhibitors were developed in the late 1990s as an alternative. They work by targeting the COX-2 enzyme, bypassing COX-1, and are therefore generally more easily tolerated from a gastrointestinal point of view. However, they turned out to increase cardiovascular risks, some more than others. In 2004, this side effect led to two of these drugs — Vioxx and Bextra — being withdrawn from the market. (For more about managing heart-related side effects, see Chapter 16.) Even though all NSAIDs can increase cardiovascular risk, at this time, Celebrex is the only COX-2 inhibitor that remains available.

Anti-inflammatories only provide symptomatic relief and are used to supplement treatment by DMARDs and immunosuppressants. Anti-inflammatories are usually taken one or more times a day. Common side effects include stomach upset, so these meds are often prescribed with stomach medications like Nexium (esomeprazole), Pantoloc (pantoprazole) or Losec (omeprazole). (For more on managing nausea and acidic stomach, see Chapter 18.)

Steroids

Corticosteroids such as prednisone and Medrol can be the best of times and the worst of times. They can be given in tablet form or as an injection in a muscle, directly in a troublesome joint or sometimes even in an IV. Steroids have decidedly beneficial effects in terms of controlling inflammation and pain and tend to work quickly. They can make you feel as if you can do anything, almost immediately giving you a strong sense of well-being. On the other hand, they can cause some pretty nasty side effects, such as weight gain, mood changes and osteoporosis (see Part II: Managing Side Effects). Prednisone is also considered by many rheumatologists as a relatively safe medication to use for pregnant women who have RA.

Steroids are usually used in one of three ways. First, they can be used to bridge the gap until a DMARD starts working. The second method is a so-called "burst," a short-term, higher dose to deal with a flare. Lastly, steroids are occasionally prescribed on a long-term basis in smaller doses, usually 5–10 mg or less daily.

Whether your treatment will include steroids depends partly on the severity of your disease and its response to the meds that are designed to suppress it. Other factors include your level of comfort with this medication and your doctor's level of comfort. Different doctors have different opinions about steroids. Some consider them a valuable tool with manageable or acceptable risks, whereas others won't prescribe them at all.

Acetominophen and Muscle Relaxants

Although NSAIDs are the most commonly used painkillers for RA, you can also use over-the-counter versions of acetaminophen and muscle relaxants.

In North America the generic name is acetaminophen — the best known brand name is Tylenol. The rest of the world calls it paracetamol. Considered a safer alternative to aspirin, acetaminophen is generally easier on the stomach and can be obtained in different strengths over-the-counter and in stronger versions by prescription. Although acetaminophen is usually well tolerated, taking too much can cause liver damage and, in some cases, acute liver failure. If you take this painkiller on a regular basis, speak to your doctor about how to do so safely.

In addition to causing inflammation in joints, RA can also affect tendons, making you use your body differently or tense up. Before you know it, not only are you battling pain in your joints, but also muscle pain. This is when muscle relaxants — officially known as skeletal muscle relaxants — can be a valuable addition to your toolkit of painkillers. They work by relaxing muscles, thereby reducing pain and stiffness. One common prescription muscle relaxant is Flexeril (cyclobenzaprine), and there are a number of others available by prescription and over-the-counter. These types of medications are commonly associated with drowsiness, so they should not be taken if you're planning to drive a car or need to focus on a task. Taking muscle relaxants before you go to bed at night allows them to work safely and can give you a better quality of sleep.

Opioids and Narcotic Painkillers

Once, years ago, I got into an altercation with my toilet that resulted in a hairline fracture in my left knee — don't ask, it's a weird and somewhat humiliating story. The pain was intense and unrelenting. It hurt when I moved, when I sat quietly and when I was lying in bed. My doctor gave me a prescription for codeine. I still remember the first time I took it. I was in bed, my knee sending out an intense pain that made my whole body feel wrong. It shrunk my world and my focus to that fracture. Then, about fifteen minutes after I took the codeine pill, I no longer cared. I realized there was still pain, but there was a wonderful cushy barrier between me and the experience of it, and I sank into the relief with extreme gratitude. I still use codeine for chronic pain, and it enables me to work, live my life and write this book. (For more on this type of drug, see Chapter 9.)

If you have a lot of pain due to uncontrolled RA or significant joint damage, it may be necessary to use opioids, also called narcotics. Opioids are classified as central nervous system depressants. They work by binding to opioid receptors, particularly in the central nervous system, as well as the gastrointestinal tract. This medication reduces or blocks the pain and can be a valuable tool in treating high levels of chronic pain.

There are a number of different kinds of opioids, ranging from medications derived from the natural source (the opium poppy) to synthetic forms of opioids created in the laboratories of pharmaceutical companies. Examples of opioids include morphine, codeine, oxycodone, fentanyl and tramadol.[26]

The primary side effects of opioids are constipation, cough suppression and respiratory depression. It's important to start slowly with these types of meds so you find out how much you can tolerate. Initially, you'll probably feel pretty woozy or sleepy and definitely should not operate heavy machinery, such as a car, until you know how you react. It shouldn't be long, though, before the medication works to control the pain without messing with your head.

There is a significant degree of concern in our world about the possibility of addiction with opioid use, and both doctors and your family and friends will probably have serious conversations with you regarding this issue. (For more on this aspect of using painkillers prescribed to treat high levels of chronic pain, see Chapter 9.)

Getting the Prescription

Many rheumatologists will tell you that they treat inflammation, not pain. This is a pretty confusing statement for those of us on the other side of the diagnosis. After all, rheumatologists specialize in treating an illness that is characterized by chronic pain. Common sense would seem to indicate that treating pain is part of treating RA, wouldn't it? Well, yes and no. If your disease is active, the pain usually originates from inflammation. Once the inflammation is suppressed, many people experience very little or no pain. Therefore, rheumatologists treat the pain of RA by treating inflammation. However, some people don't respond to DMARDs or biologics and may need stronger painkillers. Others have joint damage that causes a different kind of pain, which may also need stronger painkillers.

Although your doctor may want to focus on treating the inflammation, most are compassionate people who understand that in order to function in your daily life, you may also need pain control. Many rheumatologists will prescribe medication to address your pain, including NSAIDs and opioids, but some are not comfortable writing these sorts of prescriptions. There is an increasing understanding that pain is a complex disease that needs its own specialist, and some doctors may feel they simply don't have the appropriate training to give you the best care in terms of pain control. And then there are the rare individuals who just don't seem to get it — I have met people whose doctors proclaimed that they "don't believe in painkillers," as if pain control is a religion. Luckily, they are in the minority.

If your rheumatologist does not treat pain, you have other options. If you do not need opioids, your family doctor can be your first point of contact to get prescriptions for anti-inflammatories and other prescription painkillers. Some family doctors are also comfortable with prescribing opioids and narcotics, but if yours is not, ask for a referral to a pain management specialist. This type of specialist treats pain through a multidisciplinary approach that includes medication, exercise, meditation, biofeedback and more (see Chapter 31). If you do need opioids, your doctor may require that you sign a treatment agreement, which is a contract about how to take your medication (see Chapter 9).

Medical Marijuana

Canada and certain US states have legalized marijuana for medical purposes for people living with chronic or debilitating illnesses, such as RA. It can be useful to treat not just the pain of your illness, but also the nausea that can accompany RA or can be a side effect of some of the medications.

Medical marijuana is available in synthetic forms (e.g., Marinol or Cesamet) or you can use natural marijuana, taking it through eating, drinking, smoking or vaporizing. Although it is easier to adjust the dosage through smoking — it's effective fairly instantly and you can stop right when you feel you've had enough — this method is generally not recommended, as it carries many of the same risks as smoking cigarettes. Using a water pipe will avoid some of these risks.

In order to be able to use, buy and/or grow marijuana for medical purposes, you have to get a referral from a doctor and register with the government. Many doctors will not supervise medical marijuana use, but you may be able to find a doctor who will help you by contacting a compassion center in your area. You can also do an Internet search for the term "medical marijuana" and your city, state or province.

Non-Prescription Topical Treatments

There is a myriad of topical treatments available, and you've no doubt seen several of them advertised on TV. Whether it is Rub•A535, Biofreeze, Deep Heat, Myoflex or the alternative remedies like Tiger Balm, oregano oil or Arnica gel, you have plenty of choices. You apply the ointment to the part of your body that hurts and rub it into your skin.

Do they work? Some do. Finding the one that will work for you is a matter of trying them out. Sometimes topical treatments can work better if you wrap a particular body part in something warm after applying the ointment.

Painkillers are important, sometimes essential, in helping you control RA pain. However, effective pain management isn't just about medication — there are many other tools and tricks that can help you get more comfortable. These will be discussed in Part III: Pain Management Toolbox.

6

Financial Assistance for Medical Care and Medication

"Do I buy food or meds?"

To get the best treatment for your RA, you need a rheumatologist. For many, being able to afford medical care can be a challenge. Even if you can access medical care, some of the medications for RA can cost a fortune. Not only do you have an illness that's going to hitch a ride for the rest of your life, treating it might have you looking at winning the lottery as a reasonable way of financing it all.

Don't worry. There are places that can help you. This chapter discusses programs available in the US and Canada to assist with the cost of medical care and medication. Other countries have similar programs. If you're not in North America, speak to your doctor or your pharmacist about your options.

Medical Care

Many countries, including Canada, have a socialized healthcare system that provides access to doctors and specialists. The cost of care is either fully funded by taxes or requires only a small user fee. In the US, it's a different story. Even the changes brought about with the passing of the 2010 Affordable Care Act (the Act) have not yet guaranteed that everyone can get the care they need. This discussion of accessing healthcare therefore focuses on the United States. Keep in mind that the landscape of medical care is changing and as the Act is implemented in the future, more people will have a better chance of accessing healthcare. Stay informed. When you live with a chronic illness, you have a vested interest in being able to access healthcare. The more you know, the better your chances are.

If you do not have medical insurance, there are still options available for you to find a doctor.

The National Association of Free and Charitable Clinics has a search function on its website where you can enter your city and state or zip code and find the nearest free clinic in your area (www.nafcclinics.org /clinics/search).

The US Department of Health and Human Services maintains a listing of health centers that are federally funded, located in most cities and many rural areas. These centers provide care even if you can't afford to pay for it. The care offered is usually basic, but they should be able to assist you with ideas for finding the specialist you need. The Department of Health and Human Services also has a search function on its website where you can find a health center in your area (findahealthcenter. [hrsa.gov/Search_HCC.aspx).

Many public hospitals also offer medical care either free of charge or on a sliding scale where you pay according to your income. The website for the National Association of Public Hospitals and Health Systems has a listing of their members, and it may include a hospital in your area (www.naph.org/Main-Menu-Category/About-NAPH/About-Our-Members/Profiles.aspx). As well, teaching hospitals may also provide free or low-cost medical care.[27]

You can also discuss the situation with your doctor. There's nothing shameful about not being able to afford the high cost of tests, medication or appointments. Most doctors entered the field because they wanted to help their patients, so if you approach the issue openly, you may be able to negotiate ways of making your care more affordable. This can include your doctor using generic medications whenever possible, giving you a reduced rate if you pay for your appointment at the time of your visit and only ordering lab tests when absolutely necessary.[28]

Medication

The meds are an essential part of protecting your health and getting on with your life. Unfortunately, even the less expensive medications can add up and some RA meds, such as the biologics, cost as much as an annual salary! Even if you have insurance, copays and annual caps on meds can put a serious dent in your budget. What do you do when paying for the meds makes you more nauseated than the meds themselves?

In Canada, the provinces have publicly funded drug assistance programs available to people who experience high prescription drug costs. In Ontario for instance, the Trillium Drug Program provides assistance to people under the age of sixty-five who do not get public assistance and who do not live in a long-term care facility. People who do get public assistance receive a drug card that will fund prescription costs. As well, for people who have private health insurance, these types of publicly funded programs may assist with costs not covered by private insurers.

Applying for these drug assistance programs can be a bit of a long process, but it is definitely worth the trouble. This kind of program will pay for your prescriptions, while you pay a reasonable deductible on a regular basis, such as quarterly. How much your deductible will be is assessed through an annual renewal process.

You can access application forms for these types of programs on the website of your provincial health ministry. As well, pharmacies usually have application packages for customers who may need them, so have a chat with your pharmacist about what to do.

In the US, people who do not have insurance can access a number of different programs for help with paying for prescriptions. If you don't have coverage for prescription drugs, the Partnership for Prescription Assistance can help you find assistance programs that are both publicly and privately funded (www.pparx.org).

Another organization is NeedyMeds (www.needymeds.org). Their website has a lot of information about programs that can help you get prescription medication for yourself or your kids. They also have a discount card that may help you get up to 80% or more off the cost of prescription and over-the-counter medications, as well as medications for your pet.[29]

Rx Outreach is a nonprofit charitable organization that provides affordable generic medications for those who qualify. In order to qualify, your income has to be less than a certain amount per year, depending on how many financially dependent people are living in your home. More information is available on their website (www.rxoutreach.com).

Many chain drug stores and discount stores such as Walgreens, CVS and Walmart have programs that can help you access generic drugs at a special lower rate. Talk to the pharmacist in the store, check their website or give them a call to find out which of your medications may qualify.[30]

We often get caught up in being judgemental about big pharmaceutical companies, but it is not necessarily justified. In addition to doing the research that leads to the development of the medications that protect your health, they may also be able to help you with the cost of these meds. For instance, the Pfizer Connection to Care may help you get funding for drugs like sulfasalazine, Celebrex and Medrol (www.pfizerhelpful answers.com).

The biologics are a special case — they are new, revolutionary and very expensive. Again, the pharmaceutical companies are stepping up to make sure that people who need them are not stopped by the issue of cost. If your rheumatologist wants to prescribe one of the biologics for you, talk to them about how to access the assistance program for that particular medication. If your rheumatologist is not able to give you that information, check out the medication's dedicated website.

Copayments

Copayments are the part of the prescription drug or doctor's visit that you pay yourself and, even with insurance, they may be difficult to afford. If you have problems paying your part of the cost, you may be underinsured. There are a number of organizations that can help.

The Patient Advocate Foundation has a handy tool on their website called the National Financial Resource Guide. This is a directory of information for people living in the US who may be in need of help with housing, utilities, food and medical treatment (www.patientadvocate.org/report.php). They also have a copay relief program, and you can find more information about this on their website (www.copays.org).

The National Underinsured Resource Directory, also created by the Patient Advocate Foundation, offers services that can help you "locate valuable resources and seek alternate coverage options or methods for better reimbursement."[31] More information is available on their website (www.patientadvocate.org/help4u.php).

This chapter is by no means a complete list of the programs that can help you get the medical care and medication you need to live better with RA. To find more, talk to your pharmacist and your doctor, check Google, as well as Internet forums and communities for people living with RA and other health conditions. There is help out there. Keep looking, keep asking questions and don't give up. Getting good medical care and medication can bring you back to health and give you back your life.

7
How to Take the Meds

"Erm... pop 'em in your mouth and swallow?"

There you are, research done, loins girded, deep breath taken and decision made. You're going to take the medication your rheumatologist has recommended. You can even feel small flutterings of hope starting in the pit of your stomach. Maybe this will work and you can get your life back.

The question is, how do you take the medication? Well, take the shot, take the pill — how difficult can it be, right?

As is the case with most aspects of living with RA, there are ways of making the process easier. Whether it is dosage scheduling, minimizing side effects, choosing which biologic to take or preparing for success, you can adapt the situation to fit your needs.

Dosing Amount and Schedule

Medication should be taken as prescribed by your doctor, but before you get the prescription, there are a few things to consider.

All medications, including the DMARDs, come with a recommended dosage. This is the dose that has been found to work best in general. However, some people need to mess with it a little to make the drug work better for them.

Any time you take a medication, there's an element of uncertainty. You don't know how you're going to react to it and sometimes, your body can have a very strong objection to the drug you just took. For years, I've been very sensitive to medication, so my doctor and I have found a way to make starting a new drug less intense. In the beginning, I take half the recommended dose. Once my body is used to that, I increase the dose by a bit, take some time to adjust and then increase again. This method can be less of a shock to the system and may also reduce side effects. If you're very nervous or have a history of being sensitive to medication, talk to your doctor about trying a more gradual approach. Keep in mind that you have to balance a number of factors in making this decision, including how severely you're flaring. Priority #1 is to protect your joints and since most medications can take up to two months to really kick in, the gradual approach would probably not be a good idea if your RA is out of control.

Medications also have a recommended dosing schedule, but different people may need to take the drug on different schedules. For instance, one person will do well getting a shot of Humira every two weeks as recommended, but you may need it every ten days or every three weeks in order to effectively suppress your disease. Trial and error will show you what your body needs. Be sure to talk to your doctor about how much you can adjust on your own and when you should check with them.

Another factor to consider is when to take your first dose. Some RA meds can make you tired, ranging from feeling a bit fatigued to being completely wiped out. The first time you take a medication, try to schedule it on a weekend or before a couple of days off from work. This will give you time to lie on the couch watching mindless TV if you have a strong reaction.

Most RA meds can irritate the stomach and some are worse than others. It's still important to eat — your stomach will feel better if it has some food to digest. Before you take that first dose of the new medication, make sure you stock up on foods that are easy on the stomach and won't make you nauseated. This can include fresh fruit or vegetables — eat them raw and cold to avoid feeling queasy. Bland foods such as chicken soup, cream of wheat, white bread for toasting, crackers and bananas can also help soothe your stomach. (For more information on dealing with stomach-related side effects, see Chapters 18, 19 and 20.)

It can be a real challenge to change your routine from not taking anything but your daily multivitamin to remembering pills every day and sometimes more than once a day. Visit your local drugstore to check out their selection of pill containers that are divided into small compartments, usually arranged by day or time of day. These types of containers range from the smaller ones with just two or three small boxes to larger varieties that have boxes for meds three to four times a day for a week. Get one that has compartments for a full week and fill it up with your meds and whatever supplements you take. Put it next to your coffee maker or in another place where you'll see it every day. Not only does a pill container help you remember to take your meds, but it can also help you cope better in another way. Digging out the pill bottles every day can make you really aware of being sick and resent having to take the meds. If you put your supplements in the pill container as well, it can help you shift into the perspective that the medication is helping to keep you healthy.

Biologics: Injection vs. Infusion

When your rheumatologist talked to you about biologics, they may have given you a few choices. When it comes to the biologic medications, you can have choices in terms of specific medications or the method of administering the drug (injection versus infusion).

If there are indications that you should not take a specific biologic, it will make the decision process easier. For instance, if you have RA and multiple sclerosis, you should not take a number of the biologics, as they can affect MS (for instance, the TNF inhibitors). However, if no such considerations exist, it usually comes down to which method of getting the drug works best for you and your lifestyle.

Injectable biologics, such as Enbrel, Humira, Simponi and Cimzia, come in a pre-filled syringe or auto injector/click pen that you can use at home. This means you can give yourself the shot in the privacy of your home when it's convenient for you based on the schedule decided by you and your doctor. This is usually once a week, every two weeks or once a month. The primary hurdle with this method is getting used to injecting yourself, but your doctor or their nurse will give you some training in how to do it. You will very quickly become used to it. Some of these meds sting when injected. You can reduce this by icing the area for five minutes or so before doing the shot. If you inject in your stomach, pinching the skin hard and holding the pinch while injecting can also reduce the sting.

Biologics that are administered by infusion, such as Remicade, Orencia and Rituxan, require going to a hospital or clinic at a set schedule, such as every six weeks, then spending part of the day receiving the medication by IV. With this method, other people handle sticking sharp objects into you. As well, although you do have to take a day out of your schedule to get the infusion, there's a longer time span between each dose.

Go Low and Go Slow vs. Treat to Target

We are all different — what works well for one person may not work for another. Therefore, finding a medication that suppresses your RA, while at the same time causing minimal side effects, can take time. It's quite common to have to try more than one of the DMARDs before you find one that sufficiently suppresses your disease. This can be an incredibly frustrating experience, but recent changes in the approach to treatment can increase the chance of earlier success.

Traditionally, RA has been treated by using a sort of pyramid or ladder of treatment. Using this approach means that you'd start on milder medications first, such as NSAIDs or steroids, then move up to a drug like Plaquenil. If that didn't work, methotrexate would enter the picture, then Arava, gradually moving on to combination therapy of two or more DMARDs at a time and increasingly stronger medication. The key words were to "go low and go slow."[32] The problem with this kind of treatment is that while you're going low and slow, the RA may be galloping, and that means a significant risk of damage to the joints. If the earlier, milder medications don't work, you'll be left unprotected from RA wreaking havoc on your joints.

With the introduction of methotrexate and the biologics, there has been a sea change in treatment approaches. Instead of merely slowing down the illness, it is now possible to stop the progression, protecting you from damage and thereby allowing you to fully participate in your life. The ultimate target is now remission.

To get there, rheumatologists are adapting the model used to treat diabetes or high blood pressure. This model is called *treat to target* (sometimes *tight control*). When treating diabetes or hypertension, the goal is to reduce blood sugar or blood pressure to a certain number. During the initial period of starting medication for these conditions, the person will be monitored closely to check if the meds are reducing blood sugar or blood pressure to the desired number. Medication will be continually adjusted until the desired result has been reached.

Applying the model of tight control to treat RA means that your meds will continue to be adjusted until control of your RA has been achieved. One early study of the treat to target model compared two approaches to treatment: one in which doctors used the traditional treatment approach, prescribing whichever therapy they felt was best. In the other approach, doctors used the treat to target approach, seeing patients every three months and adjusting medications if the individuals were not in remission. After a year and a half, 18% in the first group were in remission and in the second, the treat to target group, 65% had achieved remission.[33] More recent studies have shown the same effect, emphasizing the need for continual assessment and adjustment of treatment. Using this approach leads to incredible rates of well-controlled RA. One estimate is that 40% of people living with RA can go into remission using one medication and approximately 50% need combination therapy, that is, using two or more medications together.[34] What an incredible difference!

This approach is still new and not all doctors follow this model. If you feel that you would benefit from a more aggressive approach to treatment, do some research and talk to your rheumatologist. Your doctor may have a specific strategy in mind, but if they won't budge and you're still flaring, consider getting a second opinion.

8
Remission

"How do I know the meds are working?"

This is how it was for me:

I spent much of 2004 in a bad flare, but to call it merely a "bad flare" minimizes its impact. Over my more than forty years with this disease I have had many flares, but only two horrific ones. This was the second.

The first one almost killed me when I was twelve. The 2004 flare ate my life, eroded everything I did and everything I was, a little more every day. There was a time when I thought I was dying.

I lived in this hell for eight months until on one of the first days in January 2005, my application for funding for Enbrel was finally approved. I picked up the medication at my pharmacy and at around 3 p.m., Jean, my family doctor, gave me my first shot. I went back home, had a nap and woke up two hours later a different person.

It was hard to pinpoint at first. I knew only that I felt not quite as sick as I had before I fell asleep. Every day I felt a little less sick, and then I noticed I was able to do things I hadn't done in a very long time. Leaning out over the armrest of my wheelchair without my back screaming, stretching my knee, making a cup of tea without being lost in a fog of pain. Every day more small movements came back and I reclaimed my life one millimeter at a time. It took many months for me to recover — years actually — the flare had been that bad. Eight years later I am still getting stronger, but it all started on that day in early January when I woke up and just knew the medication was working.

Defining and Measuring Remission

Remission. We talk about it, we work towards it, we dream of it, but what does it look like?

To be in remission means to have no evidence of RA activity. It's very rare for someone with RA to experience a spontaneous remission. Most of the time, remission is dependent on medications to suppress your RA. In 95% of cases the disease comes back if the medication is stopped.[35]

RA remission is measured using a combination of different factors, such as number of swollen and/or tender joints, blood test results for inflammation and the person's own report of how well they function. Currently, there are five different indices of remission and each puts a different weight on different factors. However, there's about an 80% overlap between them, so they agree on most of the measurements. At this time, rheumatologists mainly use the Disease Activity Score-28 (DAS28) to assess treatment progress. Based on this scale, low disease activity is also considered an acceptable outcome.[36]

Which measure of remission is used matters less than the approach to treatment. As discussed in Chapter 7, it's important that the treatment is started early and aggressively, using the *treat to target* model, also called *tight control*. This model of treatment keeps a close eye on your progress, re-evaluating every three months and adjusting when the meds aren't working as well as they should. By using this approach, approximately 40–50% of people with RA can go into remission and many others can get to a place where their RA is well-controlled and they have low disease activity.[37]

From the point of view of someone who lives with RA, remission can be defined in an even simpler way related to a concept called Health-Related Quality of Life. This means you have a reduction of symptoms (stiffness and pain), stopping damage and destruction in joints and improving function, which will allow you to participate in your family, at work and in your community.[38] This is the goal — for your RA to be muttering in the background instead of taking over. The goal is for you to be able to live your life again.

Coming Back to Life

Most DMARDs take a while to kick in, generally up to a couple of months. As mentioned earlier, it's quite common to have to try several different medications before you find one that works for you. But you don't have to wait two months or scour your blood test results before you start to notice a difference.

Often, one of the first signs that the medication is working is that you have more energy. It starts as a trickle, barely noticeable at first. Then one day, you realize you've made lunch and don't feel like you have to sit down for a rest afterwards.

Energy comes back first, then a small decrease in the pain, and you no longer feel as soggy and heavy when you move. One day you look at your hands and you can actually see individual knuckles instead of a puffy, swollen ridge. It can be like living within a miracle, and throughout this period of gradually getting your body back, there are moments of joy so intense that you laugh and cry at the same time.

It can also be terrifying. Once you've come out of a flare and gotten your life back, you go through your days with the awareness that a relapse is possible at any moment. I call it "living under the shoe." RA is an unpredictable disease, and when you've shared your life with it for a while, waiting for the other shoe to drop becomes part of you. A superstition develops, a reluctance to say the word "remission" for fear that it will jinx you and bring the RA back with a vengeance. Many of us will verbally turn ourselves into pretzels rather than say the R-word. Instead, we say that our RA is "managed," "under control" or "suppressed" and knock wood every time we talk about it. This fear can take over your life and make it hard to trust the medication. It may also keep you from jumping in and enjoying your life, instead spending your time being anxious and waiting for it all to go bad again. You have to find your own way through this, one step at a time, gradually adjusting to being better. At the end of the day, you have to decide whether you want to live in fear or get out there and make the most of your remission.

But What if You Don't?

There are more medications and more hope now than there ever was before, but for some, it is still not enough. Some people don't get the suppression of RA we all hope for, either because the medication isn't working or because they can't tolerate the meds without serious side effects. It is heartbreaking, devastating and can reduce your life to just getting through each day. It is a flare that doesn't stop, and there's no way of making it pretty.

Research is continuing and new medications are being developed all the time. In the past couple of years, the rate of release of new biologics has accelerated and this offers hope. The more options there are, the higher the chance that one of these medications will work for even the most stubborn case of RA.

Having faith and finding hope while RA rages out of control can be a full-time job, one that needs all the support you can find, from your doctor, from your family and from your community. If you're having trouble finding a medication that works for you, don't go through it alone.

Pain and illness isolates — in this aspect, we are very much like wild animals. The urge to crawl into a cave and lick your wounds can be overwhelming, but withdrawing only makes it harder to cope. Stay in touch with your friends and loved ones. If having visits requires too much of the energy you need to get through the day, connect by frequent phone calls. Find ways of laughing, even if it is from the deepest, darkest gallows humor. If you need to cry, do so. Releasing the sadness and despair lightens the load a little.

Online communities can be a lifesaver when you have too much pain and too little energy to go out. You check into the sites when you want and can do it in your PJs and with unwashed hair. Connecting with others in the same situation can be incredibly liberating and empowering. When you get support from somebody who's been there, it goes deeper and somehow means more. These types of communities can also you give you practical tips and advice and help you to be more informed about RA. Examples of such communities are HealthCentral's RA site (www.healthcentral.com/rheumatoid-arthritis) and RA Chicks (rachicks.com).

Both the Arthritis Foundation in the US (community.arthritis.org) and the Arthritis Society in Canada (www.arthritis.ca) have community forums on their sites, as well. If you're on Facebook, there are many different community groups there, as well.

When things get really hard, counseling can be a big help and doesn't have to be expensive. If you go to church, your pastor may be able to help you. For those who live in the US, the Partnership for Prescription Assistance has a tool on their website called the Free/Low-Cost Health Clinic Finder that may help you find a counselor (www.pparx.org/en/prescription_assistance_programs/free_clinic_finder). If you live in Canada, talk to your family doctor about mental health services in the community. Your local health department should also be able to give you some leads to access options for counseling.

Getting a referral to a pain management specialist or a pain management clinic can also be very valuable. Often, the depression that can accompany a flare can be eased by finding better ways of managing the pain. (For more on this, see Chapter 31.)

High levels of chronic stress like what is experienced during a prolonged RA flare can lead to depression, and this isn't just feelings of sadness that can be cured by watching a funny movie. Stress triggers the release of stress hormones and immune system proteins, such as interleukin-6, which can trigger depression. Trying to pull yourself up by your bootstraps is impossible when your body chemistry is set to depression. In addition to counseling, antidepressants can be a valuable tool in helping you cope. If you feel like you're drowning, have an honest conversation with your doctor about needing help.

The Future: New Criteria for Remission

In 2010, the American College of Rheumatology and the European League Against Rheumatism (ACR/EULAR) released the classification criteria for clinical trials mentioned in Chapter 1. In 2011, ACR/EULAR created a new set of remission criteria, also intended for use in clinical trials. These criteria are very stringent, specifying no more than one swollen joint and one tender joint, very low personal assessment of function on a 0-100 scale, where 0 equals very well and blood tests indicating inflammation should be very low.[39]

Several studies have shown that based on these criteria, only 6% of people with RA can be said to be in remission. That's a very difficult number to process and can make you feel very hopeless. However, when you apply these criteria to individual cases, you begin to see how this number came about. For instance, 15–20% of people who have RA also have fibromyalgia, and although such people may have no RA activity, their joints can still be tender due to the fibromyalgia. Therefore, they may not meet the ACR/EULAR criteria for remission, even though they don't have any symptoms of active RA.[40]

Both sets of ACR/EULAR criteria are bold harbingers of the future. With the classification criteria's emphasis on identifying RA in its early stages and the remission criteria's tight standards, they show where RA treatment is headed. In the future — and probably the not too distant future — the goal will be to identify and treat RA so early that remission will look like normal health. And that means there are very good reasons to hope.

9

Opiods, the Fear of Addiction and Treatment Agreements

"I don't want to become addicted."

There was a time in my life when I started every day crying in the shower. The pain was so great that I couldn't hide it, especially not straight out of bed still feeling soft and vulnerable. And so, I cried every morning. Then my doctor gave me a prescription for codeine to take as part of my regular pain management regimen and I stopped crying. This was also the start of numerous conversations with well-meaning loved ones. When I was in raptures about how effective the new meds were for my pain, they earnestly spoke to me about addiction and asked if it was really a good idea to take these pills.

RA often comes with varying degrees of pain. It's much better than it was — the changes in treatments have meant that many people who have RA don't live with significant levels of pain. In fact, thanks to better treatments many more now have their RA well enough controlled that they have no pain or entirely reasonable levels of pain. These people might be able to manage with anti-inflammatories, over-the-counter pain meds and smart use of energy.

Others need more help. Whether it is pain resulting from years of damage to joints, inability to access treatment or not being able to find a medication that works, some live with chronic, severe pain. And when you live with the kind of pain levels that keep you from leaving the house or even getting dressed, you need help to get through the day. The kind of help that comes with the Big Painkillers — Vicodin, Lortab, OxyContin and others like them. Unfortunately, this kind of help can mean that not only will your family and friends start talking about addiction, but your doctor might, too.

Opioids, opiates, narcotics — whatever you call them, these kinds of drugs do have a potential for addiction. However, the numbers are generally not as high as most people perceive them to be. One review of studies showed that when prescribed and taken correctly only *one quarter of one percent* of those taking the drugs became addicted.[41] Another review of sixty-seven studies that included patients with a history of substance abuse concluded that "the prevalence of clinically diagnosed opioid abuse or addiction was reported as 3.3 percent."[42] This means that between 96% and 99% of people taking opioids for pain **do not** get addicted, nor do they abuse pain medication. That puts a different spin on things, doesn't it?

Dependence or Addiction?

One of the factors that may contribute to the misperceptions about addiction and opioids for pain control is a lack of understanding of the difference between addiction and dependence.

Addiction is neurobiological disease. The American Society of Addiction Medicine defines addiction as "a primary, chronic disease of brain reward, motivation, memory and related circuitry."[43] This causes the addicted person to use drugs to get high instead of for pain relief. Addiction to a drug involves dysfunctional behaviors, including compulsive use, a craving for the drug and continuing to use the drug despite physical, mental or social harm.

Physical dependence or *habituation* means that your body has become used to a drug and that you may experience withdrawal if you stop taking it "cold turkey." Opioids can cause a physical dependence, but so can other non-opioid types of medication such as beta blockers and antidepressants. Even something as mundane as caffeine can cause withdrawal symptoms if you're used to drinking a lot of coffee and suddenly stop.

Your body may also develop a *tolerance* to a medication. This means that the drug is no longer as effective as it was when you first started taking it and you may need to increase the dose or switch to another drug to get good results.[44]

Aside from the physiological responses that happen within your body, people who live with chronic pain may depend on medication to be able to function. In this case, opioids can have a positive impact on your life. Taking opioids can enable you to participate in your family, work, play with your kids, walk the dog and remember what it's like to laugh every day. Just as diabetics depend on insulin to stay healthy and active, opioids can make the difference between being housebound and unable to move or being able to participate and live your life again.

What if You've Been Addicted in the Past?

If you've had problems with substance abuse in the past, it's natural to be concerned about how you'll react to opioids. The biggest risk factor for addiction to narcotics is to have a history of substance abuse. If you're in recovery, remember that the goal of your pain management strategy is the same as it is for people who have not experienced addiction: to control your pain so you can get on with your life. Having had a substance abuse problem in the past — or having one now — doesn't mean you don't deserve to have your pain treated.

Being honest with your doctor about your experience with addiction will help them tailor treatment that can protect you while giving you adequate pain control. It's important to make sure that you are not undertreated. Not having proper pain control carries the biggest risk for relapse. If you don't have adequate control of your pain, you may try to self-medicate using alcohol, other people's medications or street drugs. Having your pain managed can actually protect you against a relapse of addiction.[45]

Work with your doctor to find resources and strategies that can help you get good pain control. This can help reassure you, your loved ones and other doctors that the treatment will address your pain, while guarding against a relapse. Strategies may include having only one doctor issuing prescriptions for painkillers, getting your medications from just one pharmacy and using non-opioid medications and other pain management strategies (see Part III: Pain Management Toolbox). You and your doctor can use a trial and error method of medication to find the minimum that will keep you comfortable — not just take the edge off, but truly comfortable. Another strategy is to regularly wean off the medication under your doctor's supervision to assess pain control effectiveness.[46] Having extra support from the people in your life will also make it easier for you, so try to involve your family, friends or addiction counselor in this process.

Treatment Agreements

It is becoming increasingly common for people who need opioids for pain control to have to sign a treatment agreement, also called a drug contract. This is a contract between you and your doctor that outlines exactly how you will take your medication (dose, intervals and so on). By signing, you also usually agree to only get pain medication from one doctor and one pharmacy, as well as to undergo regular or random drug tests. Failure to follow the agreement can result in immediate termination of care — in other words being fired by your doctor. This may make it difficult for you to find another doctor who will prescribe narcotics for you.

In my opinion, the War on Drugs has lost sight of the difference between bad drugs and good drugs. This has led to a situation in which doctors who prescribe opioids are under intense scrutiny by governments and regulatory bodies to make sure they don't overprescribe medication or help addicts get controlled substances. As well, the emphasis on the potential for addiction often means that people who ask for stronger pain meds are looked at with suspicion. As I'm sure you can tell, I have strong opinions about this topic that are perhaps best shared in another format. What's important here is to give you tips on how to deal with a treatment agreement, should you encounter one. So, onwards!

Treatment agreements can be perceived as unnecessarily restrictive. Seen from another perspective, they can also help you.

Treatment agreements don't just include the specifics regarding getting prescriptions, drug tests and so on. They also outline information you need in order to have informed consent, such as details about side effects, tolerance and the (small) risk of addiction. As well, by signing and following such an agreement, you're helping to protect your doctor by providing documented proof that they have done everything they can to prevent misuse of the drugs they prescribe. This allows them to continue their practice, and that's good for you and the other people your doctor is treating for chronic pain.

If your doctor requires you to sign a treatment agreement, treat it like what it is: a legal document obliging you to follow certain rules. Make sure you read and understand it before you sign. Ask questions about a number of different scenarios, so you know how they can affect your treatment or drug test.

Ask about when you need to inform your doctor about changes that may affect how much or how little medication you take. For instance, dental work or medical procedures may involve a prescription for narcotic painkillers — do you need to tell your doctor about this? Talk about the unpredictability of RA and what to do if you have more or less pain than normal — will you be able to adjust the medication yourself as needed?

It's also a good idea to ask questions about the legislation that governs carrying opioids on your person. In some US states, you can get arrested if you carry opioids that are not in the original container labeled with your name and your doctor's name. On the other hand, carrying your entire prescription with you in the original bottle leaves you vulnerable to loss or theft. If you get robbed, you may not be able to get another prescription until your next regularly scheduled refill time. In Canada, the approach is a bit more relaxed. You may get questioned about unidentified pills, but the police will usually contact your doctor or pharmacist before considering handcuffs.[47] Ask your doctor for advice on this important issue.

Remember that it is your responsibility to keep your opioids in a safe and secure location where they cannot be accessed by anyone other than you. This ensures that you have the medication you need, while protecting others against an accidental overdose or misuse.

You also need to ask questions regarding what happens in case of a problem with your drug test. Will you have an opportunity to discuss the issue with your doctor before a decision about termination of care is made? Will you be able to have a second test to double check the results? If your doctor terminates you, will they continue to treat you for thirty days, giving you time to find another doctor? Will they give you a thirty-day supply of the medication so you don't go into withdrawal?[48]

Your doctor will probably give you a take-home package including a list of dos and don'ts and a copy of the contract. If they don't, ask for it. It's normal to forget a good portion of what happens in a medical appointment, due to anxiety and the sheer volume of information. Having something you can read through again at home can help deepen your understanding of the process and minimize the risk of problems.

When used correctly as part of quality medical care, a treatment agreement can be a tool to enhance communication between you and your doctor. A good doctor will encourage you to be honest and ask questions, making sure that you understand the agreement fully. They will put your right to effective pain control first.

Living with chronic pain requires a mental and emotional shift, not just from your doctor and the rest of the people in your life, but also from within yourself. Treating chronic pain is very different than treating acute pain and is not limited to medication (for more, see Part III: Pain Management Toolbox). However, taking medication can be a valuable part of your pain management strategy. Many people have difficulties in adapting to a different way of viewing medication, especially opioids. Try to remember that these drugs are not inherently bad. They are tools to help you get back to what's most important — your life. (For more on the approach to treating chronic pain, see Chapter 30.)

In September 2010, the first International Pain Summit was held in Montréal, Canada at the 13th World Congress on Pain. The delegates passed what has become known as the Declaration of Montréal. This declaration states that "access to pain management is a fundamental human right."[49] If you ever doubt that you really need the medication, if you ever start to wonder whether the media, your neighbor, your mother or perhaps even your doctor are right — maybe if you just tried harder, you could make the pain go away by using only your willpower — remember that statement.

It is your right to have your pain treated.

10
Medication Wrap-Up

"Can I go hide now?"

Well, that was a bit of a mouthful, wasn't it?

The world of RA meds is a daunting one, both to newbies and veterans of the disease. It's altogether tempting to stick your head in the sand and use the "I don't wanna" approach to treating your disease. Surely, there must be another way. Something that doesn't involve the meds or knowing anything about them.

For a long time, I played ostrich. I treated my RA with anti-inflammatories and it wasn't just because there were very few options available in terms of controlling my disease. I had spent my childhood and much of my adolescence immersed in JRA, hospitals and treatment (that didn't do anything), and I wanted to pretend I was normal. I was lucky — this was during a period of very low disease activity. The consequences of my denial of reality happened so slowly I didn't notice. With what I know now, I believe this was incredibly foolish. Had I sought more aggressive treatment, I might have more ability now, twenty years later. I try to be kind to my younger self and don't waste a lot of time on useless remonstrating, instead focusing on what I can do now to protect myself. Although there is still no cure for RA, we have more options than ever before.

Current treatment options are creating a reality for people living with RA that I never thought I'd see in my lifetime. I know people who kickbox, ride horses and bikes, have children, work full-time and in almost every way have completely normal lives. For most of my life with RA, much of this was not possible. Instead you deteriorated, becoming more disabled with every year that passed. Being physically active, taking care of a family, working — very little of this was possible.

Because of this changed reality, there is a shift in how you can approach your life with RA. Staying informed about the disease and the medications that treat it will help you understand what's going on in your body, the benefits of treatment and the consequences of not treating the disease. Understanding makes you engaged and empowered. It gives you a sense of control. Being informed and empowered makes a tremendous difference, even when you don't respond well to the meds that are currently available. It is the difference between being a passive passenger and taking the reins of your life.

And there's another thing. Going on the meds while fighting emotionally all the way sends a message to your emotions and your body. I'm not going to suggest that willpower has anything to do with how the meds work, but it does affect your emotional well-being. Embracing the medication and believing it is a valuable tool in your quest to get healthy will make you feel positive and hopeful. And hope is what will get you through.

PART II:
MANAGING SIDE EFFECTS

11
Side Effects from Top to Bottom

The best way we know to control RA is with medications. They come with great benefits, but also with the potential for side effects. This section of the book contains chapters on how to manage various kinds of mild and moderate side effects from RA meds like DMARDs, biologics and painkillers. It's organized starting from the top of your head and going down your body to your toes. Not that there are side effects specifically pertaining to your toes, but you get the idea.

This is not a complete list of every possible side effect there is. I discuss the side effects that are most commonly experienced or those that I've noticed people with RA tend to worry about the most. It's always a good idea to run new and/or weird symptoms by your doctor to make sure they are benign issues you can manage on your own. This will also create a record in your medical file of how you react to medication, which can be valuable information to have. Over time, these conversations with your doctor will help identify what you can shrug off and deal with yourself and what needs to be checked by a medical professional.

The tips and tricks presented in these chapters come mainly from my personal experience, learned through trial and error over the years. Some have been given to me by friends, my mother, my naturopath and my shiatsu therapist, and I'm sure I picked up a few in various magazines and websites, as well.

The information in the side effects section can be a bit overwhelming if you read it all in one sitting. Doing so might persuade you never to take another pill as long as you live! Keep in mind that it's quite likely you won't get all of these side effects, probably not even most of them. I therefore suggest that you treat this part of the book as a reference guide to potential side effects and read specific chapters as you need them.

Don't Panic

When your rheumatologist suggests that you consider a new medication, it's a good idea to do as much research as possible so you know what to expect. One possible "side effect" of this research can be a panic attack.

Like most other things we consume, medications have a whole slew of effects on the body. There are the ones they're designed to have — effects that treat a disease — and then there are the other effects that have nothing to do with the condition, a kind of collateral damage. We call these undesirables "side effects" and they can range from mild and moderate, which are often manageable, to severe and even fatal. Pharmaceutical companies are required to report every single side effect encountered during testing and after the drug has been released. Reading lists of the horrible things that might potentially happen can be enough to slam you into a fetal position, curled up and gibbering in a corner.

Relax. Not just because the odds are pretty good that you'll have entirely manageable side effects, but also because worrying about them can actually make side effects worse![50] There is a very strong link between your mind and your body, and worrying can play tricks on you, making it harder to cope.

It's also important to remember that you'll probably only have a few side effects and they'll likely be temporary or lessen over time. Some will last for a few days just after you take your medication, some will diminish and be almost unnoticeable as your body gets used to the meds and some become just another part of your life.

The reason these side effects are usually divided into *common, less common* and *rare* is because the rare — and often really scary — side effects don't happen very often. It can be a bit of a leap of faith to take a medication that you know can potentially cause serious medical conditions. Keep in mind that all medications, whether for RA, high blood pressure, diabetes or migraines, have the potential to cause rare and scary side effects. If you look at the other side of the coin, these medications can also manage your pain, protect you from having heart attacks and strokes and prevent disease-related side effects that can make life very difficult (or kill you). In the end, the benefits often outweigh the risks.

Tools and Trust

Dealing with the side effects of medications used to treat RA requires a variety of tools. Consider these chapters your toolbox filled with different doodads and ideas such as prescription medication, over-the-counter medication, supplements, foods and every now and again, certain forms of candy (no lie — I'm going to be mentioning candy). These suggestions can help you create an arsenal to minimize the experience of side effects and get the most from your medications.

When discussing supplements, I have been careful to only include those that are generally well-tolerated and which should not have any interactions with your medications. As with anything, there is an art and a skill to using supplements, the intricacies of which can be beyond lay people. I highly recommend that you consult a licensed doctor of naturopathic medicine to get expert guidance in this area. Naturopathic medicine is an alternative medicine that focuses on natural treatments from a holistic point of view, including mind and body. Treatments include herbal supplements, acupuncture, homeopathy and counseling. In the US and Canada, practitioners receive a Naturopathic Doctor degree (ND) after a four-year study at an accredited naturopathic medical school. Make sure your naturopath is properly licensed before you seek treatment. You should also discuss supplements with your family doctor or rheumatologist. Although an in-depth study of supplements and herbal medicines is usually not part of a regular medical degree, many doctors have made an effort to educate themselves in this area.

As you try different tools to manage your side effects, you'll find that some work better for you than others. That statement is becoming a kind of mantra in this book, but people react differently to medications and other tools to manage symptoms and side effects. Over time, you'll discover what works best for you. As you go along, integrating the tools in your daily routine will become second nature.

If the side effects take up too much of your life and start to limit you as much as your RA would, they may have crossed the line from manageable side effects to those that can't be managed. If this happens, it could be time to have a talk with your rheumatologist about possibly switching meds.

Trust yourself. If a small, niggling voice in the back of your head is telling you the side effects are unreasonable, listen to it. When you have RA, it's normal to often feel vaguely unwell, and this makes it easy to disappear into just soldiering through and quietly sucking up the symptoms. However, just as you need to pay attention to your body to know when it's time to ask your doctor for better treatment to control your disease, you also need to pay attention to the side effects. The goal of these medications is to enable you to get back to your life, not to feel sick in another way.

12
Fatigue and Fuzzy Brains

"I'm so tired, I don't remember my own name."

A deep desire to sleep for days. Searching for the right words and finding nothing. Feeling as if your IQ has taken a sudden plunge. These are fairly normal — and temporary — side effects of certain medications used to control RA. Usually they last only a couple of days. These kinds of side effects tend to happen especially with medications that suppress your immune system, like methotrexate or the biologics. Luckily, these medications are taken on an interval schedule, such as once a week or every two weeks, so you don't spend your entire life walking around in a pea soup fog. Your levels of fatigue and mental fuzziness will likely be in the mild to moderate range and can usually be managed without impacting your life too much.

Fatigue

You do your shot at one o'clock in the afternoon and two hours later, you're ready for a long nap. The next day you stumble out of bed, go through your morning routine like a zombie and consider getting your coffee in an IV instead of a cup. The good news is that the medication will reduce the bone-crushing fatigue that comes with flaring RA. The other good news is that as your body gets used to the medication, the drug-related fatigue usually decreases. It's unlikely to disappear completely, though, so you can count on having a couple of days after your meds of being more tired than normal.

When you first start your medication — tablets, shot or infusion — try to schedule it during a time that has a lower activity level. For instance, if you work Monday to Friday, take your meds on a Friday so you have the weekend to discover just how much of an impact they will have. Taking notes in your symptom diary (see Chapter 1) to identify the patterns of the fatigue can help you get an idea of how much you need to rearrange your life.

If your fatigue is on the milder end of the continuum, leaving you feeling as if you haven't slept well for a few days, you'll probably still be able to go to work, do chores and other tasks in your life. Working around this level of fatigue can include rearranging the tasks at work to focus on more routine activities, making double batches of meals to freeze portions for tired days and scheduling social activities for when you'll be more energetic.

If your job requires precision and focus and if you are on the moderate end of the fatigue scale, take your meds before your day off. It's likely that you will be able to mess around with your medication schedule so it works for your life, but you should consult your doctor before you do so. You may also want to ask your doctor to check your iron and vitamin B and D levels, as these types of deficiencies can contribute to fatigue. Talk to your doctor or naturopath about vitamin B12 shots — they can give you a terrific boost of energy. Other kinds of supplements may also help you get more energy, but you should consult a licensed doctor of naturopathic medicine for advice about your particular situation (see Chapter 11).

We all have lives that are becoming busier, packed to the brim with activity, and most of us long for some down time. Why not take this opportunity given to you by RA to slow the pace a little, making it a choice, as well as a necessity? Make your tired days low key, watch a good movie cuddled up on the couch with your kids and a bowl of popcorn, sleep in and delegate cooking (or heating up frozen meals) to your spouse. Consider it your gift to yourself and your family.

Living in a Fog

The meds can do a number on your mental clarity. On one hand, the difficulty focusing that comes with an active flare will ease. On the other hand, some of the drugs like methotrexate and the biologics can make your brain feel full of a thick fog, making it difficult to find words and causing you to stumble over ideas. I once saw this side effect described as confusion, but that sounds too much like I'm going senile. I prefer to call it "having a fuzzy day."

People don't talk about this particular side effect too much. We can deal with being in pain. We can even be upfront about having trouble physically doing what we used to do. But having memory issues or trouble finding the word for the big, white, cold thing in the kitchen where the milk lives? That feels embarrassing, even shameful. If you don't know what to expect, it can feel as if you're losing your mind and that is terrifying.

Thankfully, your foggy days should, like the fatigue, only last a day or two. They may vary in severity depending on what else is going on in your life, but will rarely interfere substantially with your ability to go about your business. I wouldn't recommend doing your taxes the day after you take your shot, and if you have an important meeting scheduled, you may want to push your injection time a day or two. Again, talk to your rheumatologist about how much you can play with your dosage schedule.

Pens and notepads become must-haves. On my fuzzy days, I'll be in the living room and think of something to add to my to-do list for the day. By the time I get to my desk, I'll have forgotten what it is and no amount of retracing my steps will bring it back to me. It didn't take me long to make sure that I have something to write with and write on in every room, as well as in my purse. In a pinch, I write on my hand. An unexpected benefit of this strategy for coping with a fuzzed-up mind is that by writing everything down, my life got much more organized! On days when I feel slow and useless, looking at my list of crossed-off items makes me realize I got much more done that day than I'd thought.

Most of all, don't be embarrassed. Sooner or later, we all get forgetful. Whether it's a sleep deprived new parent, a menopausal woman or just getting older, things can get foggy for the best of us. The trick is to find ways of compensating for it like carrying a pen and some Post-it notes. Let go of the part of you that feels ashamed. Getting funny about it can help. I am fond of using the term "having a blonde moment," as well as

71

telling people that I used to have a mind like a steel trap, but now it's more like a steel sieve. At the end of the day, getting it all in perspective — fuzzy mind vs. flaring RA — makes it a lot easier to accept.

13
Mood Swings and Mental Gymnastics

"I feel like Mr. Hyde..."

'Roid Rage

Tales of excessive aggression due to steroid use are normally connected to thick-necked jocks trying to build muscles on top of already bulging muscles. Such people take these drugs illegally. Those of us who live with RA take steroids entirely within the law when prednisone is prescribed to help manage the disease.

When I was about twelve years old, my juvenile rheumatoid arthritis (now called juvenile idiopathic arthritis) flared systemically, causing inflammation of my heart, spleen and other internal organs. I almost died. Prednisone saved my life, but with that came some side effects. A permanent side effect was that it stunted my growth — I look much like the Eastern European gymnasts of the past, except without the agility. The temporary side effects included a ravenous appetite and weight gain. I was eventually weaned off prednisone and these days, my steroid use is limited to the occasional shot in joints that really need them. For me and many others, steroids are miracle drugs. They give me an improved sense of well-being, increased energy and as mentioned above, make me hungry enough that I could eat everything that isn't nailed down. I have never personally experienced changes in mood.

Some do, however. In the literature about steroids, it's listed as "mental/mood changes" or "mood swings," a description that pales in the light of what can really happen. Some people experience changes to a degree that qualifies as mental instability. This can include extreme irritability, depression, hallucinations, moods that swing quickly from one end of the spectrum to the other and mistaken feelings of being mistreated. It can have an intense impact on your life, changing you from a laid-back, cheerful person to someone who makes other people nervous. It can make you nervous, too. I have friends who tell me that this shift from Dr. Jekyll to Mr. Hyde is horribly disconcerting, truly making them feel as if they are losing their minds.

One problem with mood changes can be that you don't tend to notice until it's become really bad. This could lead to spending weeks apologizing to your loved ones for your steroid-induced behavior. You may therefore want to enlist your family and friends as a safety net. Ask them to let you know if things start going south so you can discuss treatment options with your rheumatologist. You should probably suggest they do it gently, perhaps while wearing protective clothing!

Luckily, these kinds of side effects are relatively rare, but if you do start feeling as if you're growing fangs, talk to your doctor about getting off prednisone. It's important that you taper off this medication slowly, instead of stopping from one day to the next. This prevents steroid withdrawal, which can cause joint pain, fatigue, nausea, vomiting and headaches. For people who have been on steroids for a long time, stopping too quickly can actually bring about an adrenal crisis which can be life-threatening.[51]

The Sky Is Falling: My Story

I'm normally a pretty anxious person — living for over four decades with a disease that regularly yanks the rug out from under you can do that. Along with pain, swelling and difficulty moving, for me this disease has come with a profound feeling of being unsafe. When your body works against you and you never know if tomorrow is the day when the RA starts flaring again, it's hard to develop a sense of equanimity. Over the years, I've learned different tricks to manage the anxiety. These have included counseling, meditation and learning to talk myself down from a panic attack. Eventually, I stopped twitching on a daily basis.

And then I started taking Enbrel.

It took a couple of years before I found out why I felt a sense of looming dread, as if I were Chicken Little and the sky was looking unstable. Being that nervous that consistently is not fun and requires a number of different coping mechanisms. You can talk to your "safe people" — the ones you can call in the middle of the night so they can persuade you that you're not going to die. You can also try to reason your way out of the panic, bite your nails, pray, pace and so on. I tried them all. Although they might have worked in one particular instance or another, the anxiety would always come back full force. It wasn't until I switched from Enbrel to Humira that I realized my anxiety was related to the medication.

Every time I get my shot, I spend one or two days feeling nervous. When I was on Enbrel, it was administered twice a week which meant there was never time to calm down between shots. However, once I was on Humira and got my shot every two weeks, the anxiety would abate after a few days. This enabled me to make the connection. When I'm feeling fretful these days, I remember that I've just had my shot, breathe deeply and promise myself that if the anxiety is still around two days later, I'll deal with it then. When that time comes I've usually forgotten all about it and moved on with my life.

Calming Down

Emotional upset as a side effect is pretty rare. If you become unusually irritable or anxious, keeping a symptom diary can help to identify potential sources of these feelings. (See Chapter 1 for more on making a symptom diary.) When you start a new medication or you experience a new symptom that doesn't require a doctor's visit, writing down how you feel each day for three to four weeks can help you identify patterns. If you're uncharacteristically nervous and trying to figure out if there's a pattern to the fretting, keeping a diary will help you feel more in control and this in turn will make you a lot less anxious!

A simple breathing exercise can also help center and calm you. It works best if you practice it regularly throughout the day and in stressful situations:

"**Breath 1**. Take a breath in and inflate your belly as if it is filling with air. This brings your attention to the breath and away from the issue at hand. Breath [sic] out naturally.

Breath 2. On the second breath, again watch it inflate the belly. On the out breath feel your entire body relax as if it is settling into the place where you are sitting (standing or lying down)

Breath 3. Breath [sic] into the belly again, this time taking in as much air as possible without straining. Hold for a count of 3 seconds and release. Again, let go of the body as much as possible so you feel the relaxation wash over it."[52]

Another possible tool to help you calm down is Bach Rescue Remedy, a homeopathic solution made from a number of flower extracts. Available in most health food stores, Rescue Remedy comes in a number of different formats. Many homeopathic solutions are made using a small amount of alcohol. In the most commonly used type of Rescue Remedy, it's grape brandy. When you feel nervous, upset or anxious, put a drop or two on your tongue or place a few drops in a glass of water and sip it slowly. If you are a recovering alcoholic or addict, you may want to use Rescue Remedy in its alcohol-free formula or pastilles. If you're on methotrexate and your doctor recommends that you stay away from alcohol entirely, even only a few drops, this may also be a good option for you. These formulas can also be helpful if you want to use Rescue Remedy to help calm down a child.

These suggestions are only three possible ways of helping you reduce anxiety. They are intended to get you started on your own personal journey to find what works for you. There are many other techniques out there and to find them, all you have to do is be curious. Read books and magazines, talk to others and pay attention to what soothes you.

If your emotional upset interferes too much with your life, your happiness and the happiness of the people around you, and you believe it is a side effect of the meds, you have a couple of options. One is to talk to your doctor about treatment options for your RA. However, if your options are limited, you may also want to look into the possibility of counseling and/or anti-anxiety medication.

14

Sinuses

"What's with the upper respiratory infections?"

Snot-logged.

It's the only way to describe a common side effect of many of the immunosuppressant drugs, particularly the biologics. Soon after the first dose, you might begin to feel a sort of woozy pressure in your sinuses, making the world spin a little. By the next morning, when you put your face under the hot spray of the shower and then bend your head forward, it's possible that clear mucus will drain out of your nose. Theoretically. Not that this happened to me (OK, it did). Will this happen to you? Maybe, maybe not. Due to the possibility, I recommend you take the first few showers after your initial dose of a biologic alone. Save the shenanigans with a partner until you're sure you won't emit the kind of bodily fluids not conducive to romance.

The biologics seem to all share the common side effect of upper respiratory infections. This is a fancy way of saying sinus infections or sinusitis. Since biologics are immunosuppressants, you will be more vulnerable to infections in general, but why the specific emphasis on your sinuses? As far as I can tell — and this is based on personal experience, not medical research — there's something about these drugs that increases mucus production. Since your respiratory system is responsible for producing mucus, you have a sort of perfect storm happening.

The sinuses are air cavities in the cranial bones located behind the cheekbones and forehead and between the eyes. When you have a cold or a sinus infection, these areas can be sore to the touch if you poke your face with your finger. Irritants like allergens (dust, pollen, etc.) and viruses can cause inflammation in the passages of your nose, and if the bacteria in the nose somehow enter the sinus cavities, you're ripe for a sinus infection. Normally, your sinuses contain defenses against these bacteria, but if you are taking an immunosuppressant drug, it's harder to fight them off. The bacteria start festering and you end up with an upper respiratory infection, aka a sinus infection.

Recent research indicates many sinus infections disappear on their own. This is good news because the fewer antibiotics you take, the better.[53] However, when your immune system is suppressed, you may need more help. This is where prevention enters the picture.

My layperson's take on the impact of biologics on your sinuses is this:

Step 1: Increased mucus production leads to pressure and irritation in the sinuses.
Step 2: Sinuses become inflamed, making it difficult for them to drain.
Step 3: Soup of mucus is trapped along with miscellaneous bacteria.
Step 4: Festering begins, infection arrives and you feel like crap.

The goal of prevention is threefold:

1) Dilute the mucus, making it easier to drain.
2) Reduce the inflammation so mucus can drain before it becomes infected.
3) Fight the bacteria.

When I first started taking immunosuppressants, I also had to take antibiotics for sinus infections every two months or so. After a couple of years on this particular merry-go-round, I worked out a way of keeping the sinus issues down to a dull roar most of the time. It's a simple recipe — all you need to do is eat and drink three easily obtained products:

Water. The more water you drink, the more diluted the mucus gets.

Pineapple juice. In addition to vitamin C, pineapple contains an anti-inflammatory enzyme. Eating pineapple or drinking pineapple juice may help reduce the inflammation in your sinuses. In my experience, the juice works best. Start with one or two small glasses a day and work your way up, if necessary. For best results, choose the real stuff — 100% pure pineapple juice (such as the Dole brand). If it becomes too acidic for your stomach or you are diabetic, you may be able to take a supplement called bromelain which is made from pineapple extract. Remember to check with your doctor or a licensed naturopath before you take any supplements, particularly if you have other health conditions. When you take bromelain for anti-inflammatory purposes, make sure not to take it with food. The supplement can also be used to aid digestion, in which case it should be taken with food (see Chapter 21).

Garlic. Not only is garlic yummy, but it also has antibacterial properties. It may therefore help you reduce the risk of sinus infections. Eat as much as you can handle by adding garlic to pretty much anything you cook. If the people around you start complaining about the smell, tell them to eat it, too — that way they won't notice. Getting your garlic through food is preferable, but garlic pills can also be helpful. Kyolic Aged Garlic Extract has been recommended to me by my naturopath and it also comes in odorless form.[54]

If you lose the battle and develop a sinus infection, you may be able to fight it off without antibiotics by increasing your intake of water, pineapple juice and garlic. Rinsing your sinuses with salt water can also help. You can buy a saline spray in your local drugstore, but you can also use a more inexpensive solution. Mix warm water with salt and taste a drop or two to check — you want it to be salty, but not so salty that it burns. Then lie down, drip the salt water into your nostrils with a Q-tip and then blow your nose. Irrigation of your sinuses with a Neti pot may also be helpful. Look for it in health food stores or online.

Keep in mind that when your immune system is suppressed, you may not be able to win the battle of the sinuses on your own. Talk to your doctor so the two of you can decide at which point you should start antibiotics.

I've been on immunosuppressants for eleven years. As I mentioned, for the first several years, I was on antibiotics for sinus infections every other month or so. At the time of writing this book, I have been antibiotic-free, at least for sinus infections, for five years. That's not to say I haven't had sinus infections — I usually have two or three a year. I've learned to manage them, though. Will this trick of water, garlic and pineapple juice work for everyone? Probably not. But if you have a lot of sinus problems as a side effect of taking immunosuppressants, it might help reduce the number or severity of them.

15
Asthma and Allergies

"Achoo!"

In the summer of 2005, I turned into a dog. More specifically, I became a bloodhound, capable of tracking the faintest scent. You'd think this would be an interesting way to live, right? Not when most of the scents triggered asthma attacks where I felt as if my lung capacity had suddenly been cut in half. Asthma and allergies often go hand in hand and yes, my allergies went wiggy, as well. There was sneezing and wheezing no matter where I went, both inside my home and out in the world. It wasn't just limited to airborne allergens. I also started reacting to foods that had never bothered me before, limiting what I could eat. And it was all because of Enbrel — for some reason, it triggered my histamine response. It felt as if I were allergic to everything.

For some people, the biologic medications seem to poke at the histamine response, causing an increase in asthma and allergy symptoms. I was an extreme case. Most people who experience this side effect have fairly mild symptoms that last a few days and are easily managed with over-the-counter allergy medication. Others may experience a somewhat stronger response, although actually transforming into a canine like I did seems rare.

For me, the benefits of the drug still more than outweighed the side effects, and I found ways to cope with the symptoms. The experience taught me a lot of tips and tricks about living with asthma and allergies, and I share those in this chapter. Keep in mind that you will probably not need most of these. But if you do, here they are.

Airborne Irritants

Unless you live in Antarctica, it's next to impossible to avoid airborne pollen. In the spring, it seems as if all plants and trees literally pop and shoot out clouds of the stuff. It's all very pretty, but if you have allergies, going outside can make you feel awful. As spring passes into summer, the grass keeps growing and pollinating and hay fever sets in. After that comes ragweed season and in the fall, rotting leaves send out spores that can be even harder to tolerate. What's an allergic person to do?

Knowing what conditions are more likely to make you react can help you plan your day, so keep an eye on pollen counts listed on the local weather channel and on weather websites. When you can, avoid going outside on high pollen days. If you have to go out, try to work around high pollen times such as the morning of warm, dry and windy days. Wet or cooler times can be easier on your airways.

It's not just the outside world that can make you feel awful. Many who are allergic to outdoor airborne irritants also have indoor allergies, for instance to dust and dust mites. Keeping dust to a minimum by frequent vacuuming can make life easier. If you're planning to renovate, consider a change to hardwood floors or linoleum rather than carpets. It's harder for dust to accumulate on smooth surfaces.

Dust mites are tiny little critters, about 0.4 mm in length, that live in your pillows, eating your dead skin cells (yes, I know that sounds gross). About 10% of the population is allergic to dust mites.[55] If you often wake up with symptoms of allergies such as scratchy eyes, sneezing and a stuffy nose, you may be one of them. If you have asthma, this allergy could trigger symptoms. While we're talking about bedding, feather comforters and pillows can also exacerbate asthma. If your symptoms seem related to where you sleep, ask your doctor for a referral to an allergist so you can get tested. They can also give you advice on hypoallergenic bedding and techniques for protecting yourself against dust mites.

For most, over-the-counter antihistamines are enough to control allergy symptoms. If you are new to the world of antihistamines and feel overwhelmed by the massive selection, ask your doctor for a recommendation. Finding the brand that works best for your symptoms is a matter of — you've guessed it — trial and error.

Some people have trouble managing the symptoms with over-the-counter meds. In such cases, stronger versions of antihistamines may also be available by prescription. You may also want to revisit the idea of seeing an allergist to discuss whether allergy shots would be appropriate for you.

If you have trouble breathing when exposed to irritants, it's a good idea to have a chat with your doctor about what's going on and possibly get tested to see if you have asthma. If you do, you will most likely get a prescription for what's called a rescue inhaler, which can help with sudden asthma attacks. Don't leave it at home — you may not need it often, but when you do, you'll be glad it's nearby. Some people who have asthma need more than rescue medication for occasional attacks. They may benefit from medication that works to keep the lungs in better shape and prevent asthma symptoms before they start. If this is indicated for you, your doctor or allergist will be able to give you more information.

Smog can also wreck havoc on your lungs and increase your allergy symptoms. These days, it's almost impossible to escape air pollution unless you move to the country. And besides, if we all moved to the country, it would soon be polluted, as well. Carry your rescue inhaler so you can use it when the smog bothers you and check the weather channel and weather websites for smog alerts. When the air turns yellow with pollution, stay inside if possible, close the windows and turn on the air conditioning. Cooling down the house can make it much easier to breathe.

Pets

For most of us, our pets are part of the family. The idea of giving them up is impossible to contemplate except in the direst of circumstances. If you find yourself developing allergy symptoms around the four-legged, there are things you can do to manage the situation.

Clean the house often and become really good friends with your vacuum cleaner — it's one of the best tools to get rid of hair and dander. Make sure your pets are clean and frequently brushed and keep the furry ones off the bed and other furniture to prevent pet dander from building up.

It you have a cat, stay away from clumping cat litters, because the dust can bother your lungs. Instead, choose cat litter made from crystals, newspaper or corn. If you don't have that option in your area, get cat litter that is advertised as being "dust-free" or "non-tracking." Getting the unscented cat litter can also help manage your symptoms.

If despite all efforts you're still itching and sneezing, over-the-counter allergy medications may be enough to solve the problem. You can also talk to your doctor about prescription allergy meds or allergy shots.

If you don't have a pet and want one, look into so-called "nonallergenic" breeds. Although there isn't such a thing as a completely hypoallergenic animal, dogs that don't shed, such as poodles and Portuguese water dogs, are less likely to cause allergic responses. As well, even though you may be allergic to cats in general, some people can get used to a specific feline friend. Living with a cat can accustom your body to that particular animal, which means you don't experience symptoms around it. Just don't give it a bath, as water tends to exacerbate the allergens. Knowing cats, it would probably also fight you tooth and nail to get out of the bath, so staying away from that idea will save you from being scratched and having to apologize. Luckily, cats are very good at keeping themselves clean.

Fragrance and Fumes

We live in a highly scented world. Almost everything — candles, lotion, detergent, even diapers — has added fragrance to make it smell nice. No matter how pleasant the smell, scent can trigger an asthma attack or a sneezing fit in people who are sensitive to fragrance.

If you're one of them, you can switch to fragrance-free soap, lotion, cleaning products, detergent and fabric softener. Luckily, these types of products are becoming much easier to find as they are also kinder to the environment. Most green or eco-friendly products are scent-free and free of chemicals. Certain products like fragrance-free shampoo and other hair products can be difficult to find in your local store, but doing a search online will help you find places that sell them. You may also be able to tolerate a regular mild shampoo. I use Johnson's baby shampoo — it has a scent, but it's mild and doesn't stay in my hair.

There's a difference between unscented and fragrance-free. Unscented means there are no added perfumes, but materials in the product may still be scented. I know that doesn't make any sense, but just go with it and don't try to apply logic! However, if the product specifically says fragrance-free, it will usually be without fragrance. Not always, though — occasionally, a small amount of fragrance may be added to cover the smell of other ingredients. Your best option is to sniff your way to a product that works for you.

If you have asthma, invest in a box of alcohol swabs. If you inject yourself with RA meds, you may already have them on hand. When I first started having trouble with scent, just shaking hands with someone who wore scented lotion would send me into a fit of wheezing. I tried washing with soap and even fresh lemon, but nothing got rid of scents in a reliable way. Later, I discovered that nothing removes a scent from your skin or an area in your house faster than wiping it with an alcohol swab.

As awareness of asthma and allergies increases, more and more workplaces are developing scent-free workplace policies. If other people's scented products affect your health at work, talk to staff in the human resources or equal opportunity department about solutions.

And then there are fumes. Just as some people are sensitive to fragrance, they may also have a reaction to fumes from a variety of sources.

Some products, such as computers, carpets and furniture, "off-gas." This is the evaporation of synthetic compounds that are used in the making of the product. Sometimes it's very noticeable — the "new car" or "new carpet" smell — and sometimes it's less obvious. If you are sensitive to off-gassing, it may help to place the product in an open area such as a balcony, basement or in front of a window for a couple of days before you use it. You may also try to talk to the staff in the store where you buy the product about letting it off-gas in their warehouse for a few days before delivery.

Paint and varnish also have strong fumes. Water-based products generally have less serious fumes that evaporate more quickly than oil-based paints and varnishes. There are also an increasing number of paint brands that are low VOC. VOC stands for Volatile Organic Compounds, which are contained in the solvent used in paint and released as the paint dries. These are the compounds that can cause reactions such as headache, nausea and difficulty breathing. Using low-VOC brands can make painting your house a healthier experience for you and the environment, too. Talk to your hardware store staff about your options.

Food Allergies and Sensitivities

For as long as I can remember, I've been sensitive to apples and grapes — when I eat too many, I get hives. When I started Enbrel in 2005, more foods joined the list.

There are roughly two kinds of reactions to food. The milder one expresses itself with hives, itching, sneezing and so on. The second — and much stronger reaction — can bring on anaphylactic shock, a potentially fatal reaction where the mouth and throat swell so much you can't breathe. This is the kind of reaction that causes schools to ban peanut butter to protect allergic children.

Although anaphylactic reactions get quite a bit of attention — deservedly so due to their seriousness — they are fairly rare. However, if you notice a reaction that involves a feeling of swelling in the lips, mouth or throat, call 911. Anaphylaxis can go from minor to scary very fast, so don't wait to see if it will go away. If you do get diagnosed with this kind of allergy, your doctor will prescribe an EpiPen that you should always carry with you. It can save your life. For more information about food allergies in general and anaphylaxis in particular, see the Food Allergy and Anaphylaxis Network in the US (www.foodallergy.org) or Anaphylaxis Canada north of the border (www.anaphylaxis.ca).

There. Now that we're all good and scared, let's move on. This is probably a good time for a reminder that should you develop a sensitivity to certain foods, it will probably be more of an irritant. If that happens, talk to your doctor about a referral to an allergist.

Managing sensitivities and allergies to different foods has a lot to do with reading labels. Labels will tell you almost everything you need to know. Some countries legally mandate that manufacturers clearly state the presence of potential allergens on the label of their food products. In addition to the regular ingredient list, some of the most common allergens such as soy, wheat, nuts, peanuts, eggs, sesame and dairy may be listed at the end of the ingredient list. When that happens, it's usually in bold type or described, such as "may contain traces of tree nuts." Shopping can become unexpectedly amusing when you find such a mention on a box of pecan cookies. To find out how much you can trust the label, look into what kind of food labeling is mandated in your area.

If your area does not require listing common allergens, you can contact the manufacturer to ask about the risk of certain allergens. Check the package for a website or do an Internet search for the product or company that makes it. Websites usually have a "contact us" area and in my experience, companies take allergy questions seriously. They don't want to inadvertently kill someone. It's bad PR.

You can also take a look at the other products made by the company. For instance, say you're allergic to nuts and want to buy a box of crackers. You look at some of the products made by the same company and find that they also make chocolate chip cookies with nuts. This could be an indication that the two products are made in the same factory and there may therefore be a risk of cross-contamination. In such a case, you should check with the company before eating the crackers.

There are also many websites and online forums related to food allergies. Those that are run by parents of allergic children can be particularly helpful. They are terrific sources of where to find safe foods and the members are very helpful.

As our world becomes more polluted, allergies and asthma are on the rise and each year, more people have to find a way to live with these health conditions. That's sort of good in a weird way, because you're not alone. Others are much more likely to understand the challenges of allergies and asthma than what it's like to live with RA.

If you develop symptoms of allergies and asthma that are strong enough to be unmanageable, and you believe they are a side effect of your medications, talk to your doctor about changing meds. Although one type of RA medication might aggravate allergies and asthma, another might not. After two years on Enbrel, I switched to Humira and my allergies and asthma subsided significantly. They're still around, especially for a couple of days after I get my shot, but I no longer feel like a tracker dog.

16

Hypertension, Strokes and Heart Attacks

"My blood pressure's through the roof!"

The summer of 2004 hadn't been nice to me, piling a ridiculous amount of stress into my life. In return, I hadn't been particularly nice to other people, growling at everyone I knew. I'd also been fighting a headache for just about the same amount of time, but chalked it and the uncharacteristic surliness up to stress. I was doing my best to deal with it so I could return to my normal life and a sunnier disposition, but wasn't being very successful. Then one day I saw a new doctor and they took my blood pressure as part of the routine workup. And it was 176/131 instead of my normal 120/70.

Not coincidentally, I was on Vioxx at the time. Vioxx was a COX-2 inhibitor, a type of nonsteroidal anti-inflammatory drug (NSAID) akin to Celebrex (see Chapter 5). A few months after I was diagnosed with high blood pressure, Merck, the makers of Vioxx, removed the drug from the market due to its side effects of increasing the risk of heart attack and stroke. All NSAIDs have the potential for these side effects, but studies indicated that the probability for someone taking Vioxx was four times higher than when taking naproxen, another NSAID (0.4% versus 0.1%).[56]

If left untreated, hypertension (high blood pressure) can lead to strokes. Some people, like me, experience symptoms when their blood pressure starts to rise, but most don't. This which is why it's sometimes called "the silent killer." If your meds carry the risk of hypertension, it's especially important to get your blood pressure checked on a regular basis. Some people buy their own blood pressure device, but if you don't have high blood pressure, there is probably no need for it — chances are it'll just make you nervous, which might increase your blood pressure!

When you have RA, you have more frequent doctor visits, so asking the doctor or nurse practitioner to take your blood pressure should be enough to keep an eye on things. This way, you'll also be aware of what your normal blood pressure is and therefore know when to talk to your doctor about possible changes in these numbers.

Should you develop high blood pressure — and most of us do as we age, whether we're on RA meds or not — it can usually be treated effectively with medication. If you have hypertension, it may be helpful for you to have your own blood pressure device, as it can be a valuable tool in assessing how you respond to medication. It may also be useful in helping you identify triggers for increased blood pressure, which can help you manage the condition. Ask your doctor to recommend which device is best and for guidance in how to use it.

Although there seems to be some debate about the role of sodium in hypertension, many people have this connection and experience a rise in blood pressure when they have too much salt. Most of us consume too much salt as it is, so it's probably a good idea to reduce your sodium intake.

It's also important to remember that certain supplements may not be appropriate for you if you have high blood pressure. Talk to your family doctor or consult a licensed naturopath to find out more about which supplements are safe for you.

Managing the risk of heart attack and stroke associated with RA and certain medications has a lot to do with prevention. Monitoring your heart health, being aware of the risk factors and working with your doctor to reduce them are the most important things you can do to lower your risk. As mentioned in Chapter 3, treating your RA is also an essential tool in lowering the risk of stroke and heart attack.

Sometimes despite all our efforts — and whether we take NSAIDs or not — a stroke or heart attack may occur. It's important that you know the signs and what to do in such a situation. Quick intervention can save your life and reduce the impact of such an event.

The Heart and Stroke Foundation of Canada lists five signs of stroke:[57]

1. Weakness. Sudden loss of strength or numbness in the face, arm or leg.
2. Trouble speaking. Sudden difficulty in speaking or understanding or sudden confusion.
3. Vision problems. Sudden trouble with vision.
4. Headache. Sudden severe and unusual headache.
5. Dizziness. Sudden loss of balance, especially combined with any of the above signs.

Strokes can be treated and the sooner you see a doctor after having a stroke, the greater the chances of minimizing its effects. If you experience any of these symptoms, call 911 immediately.

Signs of heart attack include:[58]

1. Pain. Sudden pain or discomfort that can feel like burning, squeezing, heaviness, tightness or pressure in the chest, neck, jaw, shoulder, arms or back.
2. Shortness of breath or difficulty breathing.
3. Nausea, indigestion or vomiting.
4. Sweating with cold or clammy skin.
5. Fear.

Although the most common symptom of heart attack for both men and women is chest pain, you should know that women may experience symptoms that are milder and more vague, as well as more gastro-intestinal. If you're a woman, talk to your doctor about this issue so you know when to act.

If you think you may be having a heart attack, call 911. Do not try to drive yourself to the hospital or take a cab. If things get bad suddenly, paramedics will be able to save your life, but a cab driver won't. Driving yourself to the hospital could also put others at risk. Should the symptoms worsen or cause you to lose consciousness, you may cause an accident.

If you're feeling scared right now, take a deep breath. Although some RA meds carry the risk of heart attack and stroke, they are in the rare side effect category. The chances of you keeling over as a result of taking these medications should be minimal.

It's the unfortunate reality that many of us get high blood pressure and will have heart attacks and strokes as we grow older, regardless of what medications we're on. However, it's also a reality that RA itself can be a risk factor for these conditions (see Chapter 3). Talk to your doctor about the risk factors and how to minimize them. Then think about the consequences of not taking the meds. It's a balance, but with your doctor's help, one that's possible to achieve.

17
Managing Infection Risk

"Do I have to live in a bubble?"

So there you are, having a cup of tea after the latest visit to your rheumatologist, pondering their recommendation that you start an immunosuppressant like methotrexate or the biologics to treat your RA. Visions of the boy in the bubble — any boy in any bubble, really — are bouncing through your mind. As you glance around you, every other person in the coffee shop starts to look as if they're enveloped in their very own cloud of germs.

What will this mean for your life? How do you manage the increased risk of infection? How scared should you be? Will you need to wear a mask when you're out in public? What will that do to your social life? Should you invest in gallons of hand sanitizer?

The answer is that you don't have to be that scared, but you shouldn't be lackadaisical either.

Several Christmases ago, my sister's then three-year-old twins came to the celebrations with an extra gift: a massive cold at the exact stage when bodily fluids are flying every five minutes. At the time, they were too young to understand the "sleeve sneeze," where you sneeze into your elbow to minimize the spread of illness. Instead, they sprayed the collected family with cold germs every time they went *achoo*. Which was often. They were also young enough to hug everybody all the time. It was like biological warfare encapsulated in two tiny and adorable Weapons of Mass Destruction. By the fifth time I was sneezed on in about thirty minutes, I gave up and resigned myself to being sick by New Year's. I mentally rearranged my injection schedule of Humira (one of the biologic drugs) to avoid giving my immune system an extra dip and hoped that would prevent me from getting really sick. Yet somehow, I stayed healthy and didn't catch their cold. Given my suppressed immune system, I have no idea how I avoided the contagion, but took it as an extra special present from a universe infected (!) with the Christmas spirit.

In the summer of 2009, a woman was at a dog show and, in the middle of a hectic day, one of the dogs accidentally clawed her leg, pulling off a piece of skin.[59] "No big deal," the woman thought. She cleaned it thoroughly, slapped a bandage on it and moved on with her day. If you're a pet owner, you know this one — there are going to be scratches and most of the time, you don't remember when you got them. So, no big deal, right?

In this case, it actually became a big deal. Because the woman was on Enbrel, her immune system was suppressed. In less than a day, she developed cellulitis, an infection of the skin and underlying tissue. This was followed by IV antibiotics, debridement (removal of dead skin), skin grafts, a hospital stay, weeks on crutches and a complete derailment of her life for several months.

Most of the time, managing infection risk is pretty easy. Staying safe does mean being alert and aware of risk factors in your environment. As well, you should also talk to your family and friends about how they can help protect you from infection. They may roll their eyes and mutter about you being paranoid, but you aren't. A scratch from your pet may heal normally and that cold that's going around may just give you the sniffles for a couple of weeks. Although it's rare, they might also trigger a domino effect in your body, causing serious and scary infections. Keeping yourself healthy takes some diligence and is a team effort between you and the people with whom you share your life.

There is no need to get rid of your pets or freak out if you get a cold, but pay attention and don't ignore signs that your body is having a hard time managing. If you don't feel right, if it feels as if something rips in your chest when you cough or if that scratch from playing with your cat gets red and starts spreading, see a doctor. If your doctor can't see you right away, go to an urgent care center or ER and explain that you're on an immunosuppressant.

One last note about animals — if you do get bitten and it breaks the skin, go to the ER immediately for IV antibiotics. Cats and dogs have germ-ridden mouths and people with perfectly healthy immune systems frequently get nasty infections from animal bites. Don't mess around with this one. Be safe.

Immunosuppressants can suppress your RA and give you back your life when nothing else helps, but really big drugs for really big problems also come with the potential for really big side effects. These medications are tools that come with a sharp edge. Just as you're careful not to chop off your fingers when you cut vegetables with an extra sharp knife, you need to be careful with these drugs. Treat them with the respect they deserve and then move on with your life.

An Ounce of Prevention

The best way to prevent getting an infection is to avoid all harmful germs and not get sick in the first place. Unless you stay in a sterile environment, that's impossible. The point of taking immunosuppressants for your RA is to get your life back and that means getting out there and *living*. You can't avoid getting sick every now and again, but there are things you can do to decrease the risk.

If you can feel yourself getting sick, or you've been exposed to somebody who's in the highly contagious stage of an illness, you may want to skip your dose of medication. If you take it, your suppressed immune system might be even more suppressed, making it harder for you to fight an illness. Ask your rheumatologist what they recommend. Some doctors suggest that you don't skip the dose unless you have a fever, while others believe you should skip the dose either way. You should also make sure to talk about the procedure for this. Some doctors like you to call and let them know and others leave the judgment of whether or not to skip the treatment up to you.

When you feel like you're about to be hit by an illness, *do not* take an immune system booster such as echinacea or goldenseal. Immune system boosters can cause autoimmune diseases to flare.[60] In illnesses such as RA, the immune system is attacking itself and if you boost the immune system to defend against the cold, you also boost that attack, thereby causing a flare.

As you can imagine, it is also a good idea to stay away from people who have a contagious illness whenever possible. This means training your family and friends to cancel plans if they're sick or have been exposed to a contagious illness within a few days of seeing you. It might take a while — people often don't understand the consequences of being immunosuppressed and some even get offended. Do as much educating as you can in terms of telling them exactly what the medication does to your system. You may also want to collect a few horror stories from the Internet to share, if necessary.

Avoid children. I say that with tongue firmly planted in cheek, but the reality is that children are germ factories. Their immune systems are new and it's their job to develop resistance to germs as they grow. Unfortunately, the only way to do this is to catch every virus going around and live through it. This way, they'll have a resistance the next time the virus goes around. If you're around a lot of children — by, for instance, working in a school — you're going to be at risk for catching whatever they have. You may be able to manage by being diligent in your use of hand sanitizer or other coping strategies (see below for suggestions). However, if you're sick all the time, talk to your rheumatologist about options. I have spoken to people who've had to change jobs, which is a great pity. But at the end of the day, it's important to stay as healthy as possible.

Buy a box of surgical masks as a "just in case" precaution for the times when you can't avoid being around people who are sick. If your mother-in-law insists on coming over despite a hacking cough, hand her a mask or wear one yourself. If you're traveling by plane — think tin can with nowhere for the germs to go — consider bringing a mask and explaining to your seatmates that you have a suppressed immune system. You might get some odd looks, but it's better than getting sick.

Having a box of medical examination gloves on hand can also help reduce the risk of contagion. You can get them in most pharmacies and drug stores, but try to avoid the latex variety to protect those who have latex allergies. Use the gloves if you're dealing with something germ-laden, like picking up dog poop in the backyard, scooping the cat litter, changing diapers, repotting plants and other types of gardening.

It's also a good idea to have a chat with your doctor about vaccinations for various infectious diseases, such as the annual flu shot and pneumonia vaccine. Also keep your tetanus shot up-to-date. Be aware that certain medications, especially the biologics, mean that you *must not* receive a live vaccine — your suppressed immune system makes it more likely that you'll develop the illness contained in the vaccine. Some also say that people with RA should not receive live vaccines at all, regardless of whether they're on biologics, as our immune systems may not be strong enough to fight off a live virus. Ask your rheumatologist for guidance.

The kitchen is home to many different kinds of bacteria. Raw ingredients, such as meat and fish, and leftover soil on vegetables can expose you to germs you might not expect. Be careful with raw meat and fish, keeping them in one area and cleaning it thoroughly with soap after you've finished. Don't rinse your chicken under the tap and then carry the pieces to the stove, dripping along the counter or floor. Make sure that utensils, cutting boards and anything else that comes into contact with food is clean. It may also be a good idea to have separate cutting boards for meat, fish and vegetables. This reduces the risk of cross-contamination, a process in which different substances can interact and create a higher risk for infection.

It's easier to control your environment in your home, but being out in public carries a whole other level of exposure to other people's germs. You can't avoid being breathed on in a crowd, but try to limit how much you touch things that are used by a lot of people. A recent study examined which public surfaces were the dirtiest. The top four were gas pump handles, handles on mailboxes, escalator rails and ATM buttons — the kind of surfaces that don't get washed daily (or ever).[61] When you do have to interact with such things, find ways of not touching them directly. Use a key, pen or cover your finger with a tissue to press elevator buttons and enter information on a debit card keypad. If a door has a button for an automatic door opener, use it. Not only will it help reduce the chances of you picking up an illness, but the joints in your hands and arms will thank you for it. When it's cold and you're wearing gloves, don't take them off until you're inside a building. Have a specific pair of gloves in your car for pumping gas and use your own pen to sign credit card receipts. You get the point. The more you stay away from surfaces touched by throngs of people, the more protected you will be.

In smaller groups or one-on-one situations, don't shake hands if you can avoid it. It took me a long time to learn this one — after all, it's instinctive to stick your hand out for a shake when you meet someone. However, after having suffered the consequences of many a good, firm handshake, I now wave, hug (friends, not strangers) or quickly explain that I don't shake hands because it hurts. I try not mention the immunosuppressed thing — it makes people feel as if I don't trust their hygiene! If your RA is not visible and you don't want to tell a stranger about your disease, a casual "I'm recovering from a sprained wrist" may do the trick. If all else fails, carry a small bottle of hand sanitizer. Thanks to the SARS virus and H1N1 flu, many perfectly healthy people carry hand sanitizer these days, so you're much less likely to offend if you use it than you were in the past. It's become just part of what people do to stay healthy.

There are a couple of things you can do to improve your general health that can also help you fight off infections. If you're a smoker, quit. The healthier your lungs are, the better able you'll be to fight possible infections. Talk to your doctor if you need help with kicking the habit. Getting enough sleep is also an important factor in helping your body stay strong. Sleep is the time when the body regenerates itself. If you have trouble sleeping because of high pain levels, speak to your doctor about better pain control (also see Part III: Pain Management Toolbox).

Much of taking care of your body and avoiding infection risk involves using common sense, as well as a certain level of assertiveness. Putting your own health first isn't easy when doing so involves potentially inconveniencing others. Your family and friends may be upset that you're canceling getting together yet again — after all, it's just a case of the sniffles, so what's the big deal? To healthy people, a slight cold is an inconvenience that doesn't stop them from doing what they need to do in their lives. To you, it can mean getting really sick, sending you to bed for days or maybe even weeks.

The more you know about your body and its reactions, as well as your RA and the implications of being immunosuppressed, the better you'll be able to educate the people in your life about the possible consequences of you getting sick. It may take a while for them to understand that you're protecting yourself against real, not imagined, risk, but over time, they'll get there and come to respect your choices.

There are times when you can't duck out of a social event even though a family member is sick and there are times when despite precautions, you'll catch something somewhere. If you do get sick, trust your gut when judging if your body is having trouble fighting back. If your cold feels like it's getting out of control, lasts a long time or you're running a fever, see your doctor. If you have trouble breathing or your cough sounds like a car that won't start, go to the ER to get checked for pneumonia. If a scratch looks infected, don't just deal with it yourself, see a medical professional. You are the best judge of your health — if you feel wrong, get checked out.

Reading information like this can convince you that your best option is to avoid immunosuppressants like the plague. As discussed in Chapter 3, the consequences of not treating your disease are significant. RA is an autoimmune disease and that means some of the best treatments currently available suppress your immune system. Any time you make a decision to treat a medical condition, there will be risks and benefits. Most of the time, the benefits of treating your RA will outweigh the potential risks. When it comes to managing the risk of infection, taking reasonable and fairly easy precautions will usually be enough to help you get back to your life.

18
Nausea and Acid

"I feel queasy and the heartburn's killing me."

The server has just put down a plate of deep-fried calamari in front of me, and as I look at it, I begin to realize that I won't be eating it after all. What was one of my favorite meals a week ago now looks greasy, smells off and when I taste one of the lightly battered pieces — I always go for the tiny whole ones first because I like the way the tentacles tickle my tongue — it tastes weird. For a moment, I feel like telling my plate, "it's not you, it's me." Because it *is* me — it's the day after my shot of Humira. The next couple of days are going to be like this — food tasting weird, so much gas I feel blown up like a balloon and don't get me started on the issue of acid! RA meds are notorious for being hard on the stomach, making you nauseated one moment and "enjoying" the flames of heartburn and bubbling stomach acid the next. There are times when it feels as if your stomach is trying to eat itself.

The first step to reduce these side effects is to listen to your pharmacist when you pick up your prescription. If they say that your NSAIDs need to be taken with food, take them with food. The traditional NSAIDs like naproxen can burn going down, and one of their nastier side effects is a higher risk of gastrointestinal bleeding. Taking the medication with food can help manage this risk.

You may also want to talk to your rheumatologist about other types of NSAIDs. Vimovo is a drug that contains both esomeprazole (see below for more about this stomach medication) and naproxen and might therefore be easier on your stomach. As well, alternative anti-inflammatories called COX-2 inhibitors (Celebrex) were developed relatively recently, but they carry their own risk factors. You may remember when Vioxx, one of the more popular COX-2 inhibitors, was recalled in 2004 due to concerns over the increased risk of heart attack and stroke (see Chapter 16). Stay informed and keep the lines of communication open with your doctor so you're aware of the costs and benefits of taking these drugs.

Medications like methotrexate and the biologics also tend to come with stomach-related side effects, especially for a few days after you take your dose. Luckily, you have several options in your toolbox that, separately and together, can take you from clenched teeth and a burning hole where your stomach used to be to getting on with your day.

Prescription Medications

Depending on the severity of your symptoms, you may want to talk to your doctor about prescription medications to reduce heartburn and gastroesophageal reflux disease (GERD). Such medications are called proton-pump inhibitors (PPIs) and decrease the amount of acid in your stomach.[62] Examples of PPIs include Losec and Prilosec (omeprazole), Nexium (esomeprazole) and Pantoloc (pantoprazole). These types of drugs are usually taken once a day, but for some people this may not be enough. Twelve hours into the day, they start feeling the acid again, but because they have to wait until the next day to take another pill, they never get ahead and continue to battle acidic stomach. If this sounds like you, ask your doctor about trying a prescription of a milder version of the stomach meds twice a day instead of a stronger one once a day. This may be more effective in keeping the acid down.

Over-the-Counter Medications

Antacids such as Gaviscon, Maalox and TUMS can be very helpful when your stomach burbles up some acid. They have different flavors, but if your heartburn is accompanied by nausea, sweet flavors like butterscotch can make things worse. Start with mint, but keep in mind that some brands add more peppermint than others and too much mint can burn, as well. Try different flavors and brands until you find one that works for you.

Gravol can also be helpful if things are really bad. You may want to try Gravol Ginger, as ginger is a terrific way of soothing the savage beast that can live in your stomach (more on ginger below).

Probiotics

Years ago, my naturopath gave me acidophilus to help heal the damage done to my stomach after decades of RA meds and painkillers. Acidophilus (a type of probiotic) is a natural bacteria that helps your digestive system. In the past it was primarily recommended when taking antibiotics, because they can destroy the natural bacteria culture in your gut. Taking acidophilus can help rebuild the natural bacteria. Recently, probiotics are enjoying a bit of an upswing, being added to milk, yogurt and other products with claims of helping your digestive system. Many, including myself, find that probiotics are also very successful in reducing the amount of stomach acid and heartburn.

Get the good stuff from the health food store, remember to keep it refrigerated and take one or two doses a day with meals. My naturopath told me that acidophilus will either help you or do nothing. It doesn't seem to have any side effects, except the possibility of loose stool if you're taking too much. If your bowel movements get loose, reducing the dose should take care of it.

Tricks with Food

If you experience problems with acid, an empty stomach can make the problem worse. It can feel almost as if your stomach is trying to eat itself. Instead of sticking to three larger meals a day, try eating frequent small meals. Between meals, snack on fresh fruit and vegetables, nuts, raisins or dry crackers. By consistently grazing as you go through your day, you're keeping your stomach busy digesting small amounts of food. This means it won't get antsy and start looking around for something to get at, attacking your stomach lining in the process.

On days when you're nauseated, stick to blander foods like baked chicken or fish. For instance, try a mild fish like sole, tilapia, cod or haddock. Steam the fish with a whole green onion and two or three whole, peeled garlic cloves — they add a slightly nutty taste without the bite of chopped garlic. Serve with rice or boiled potatoes for a meal that's easier for your stomach to handle when you're feeling queasy.

Fresh fruit and vegetables are also easier to handle when your stomach's cranky. Staying away from rich, fried and spicy foods can ease the protests from your mid-region. Reducing the amount of sugar in your diet may also be helpful. Sweet foods and treats can get the acid going and trigger nausea, as well.

As I've mentioned before, ginger can be a terrific tool in reducing nausea. A 2009 study by the National Cancer Institute found that ginger was helpful in reducing the nausea that accompanies chemotherapy.[63] It is usually well tolerated, but may cause heartburn if you take too much. Start with a small amount until you find what works best. You should be aware that ginger can bump your blood pressure a bit, so if you have hypertension, be sure to keep an eye on this. Adding ginger to your life is easy. You can use ginger in your recipes — it adds a lovely flavor to almost anything. Buy some fresh ginger root at the supermarket, peel the skin off, then slice, chop or grate the piece and add it as you cook. Ginger chews (candy) and ginger capsules can also help, and both are usually available in health food stores. Gravol Ginger contains ginger root and can be found in your local drugstore. It does not, however, contain the anti-nausea medication in regular Gravol.

Hot Drinks

Coffee, tea and other caffeinated beverages can be murder on your stomach, but there are a number of other possibilities for hot drinks. Decaffeinated coffee and tea are gentler if you can't make it through the day without their flavor, but other types of herbal teas may be more effective. Peppermint tea can do wonders when you're queasy, and ginger tea is also a terrific, natural way of soothing an upset stomach.

If you buy ginger tea, make sure it's made with real ginger root instead of ginger flavoring. Ginger tea is also easy to make yourself. Get a piece of fresh ginger and cut off a small slice — about the size of a nickel or so for one cup or a larger piece if you're making a pot. Peel the piece and let it steep in boiling water for ten to fifteen minutes. Add a small squeeze of lemon for flavoring or a bit of honey if you prefer.

And speaking of lemon. Years ago, my shiatsu therapist recommended hot water with a small slice of lemon for my stomach problems. Although it sounds strange to add lemon to an acidic stomach, it does help me. I was told it works on a sort of homeopathic principle — a little of what hurts you can be helpful. Be conservative in your approach until you discover how much is right for you. Cut a fairly thin slice of lemon and then cut it again into three or four pieces. Add one piece to a mug of hot water and enjoy! Not only does it soothe your stomach, it is also wonderfully refreshing and can help you drink more water.

Acupressure

There's an acupressure point on the inside of your wrist that when pressed, may help you feel less nauseated. Acupressure follows the same principles as acupuncture, but applies pressure instead of inserting needles. (For more on acupuncture, see Chapter 33.) There is a product called Sea-Band that is used to relieve motion sickness. It's a sort of bracelet that is worn on your wrist with a small pellet or marble at the acupressure point for nausea relief. Sea-Bands are usually available in larger drugstores.

Vomiting

The queasiness that may come with RA meds can often be managed with the tips listed above. For most, it rarely progresses to actual vomiting. Should you start throwing up, treat it like you would a stomach bug. Drink as much as you can to make sure you don't get dehydrated. Warm water with lemon or weak ginger tea can be very soothing and may reduce the nausea. You can also take anti-nausea medication, such as Gravol or Gravol Ginger. Again, be aware that Gravol Ginger contains only ginger root, not anti-nausea medication.

If the vomiting continues, check in with your family doctor. It may be a sign that you have a stomach bug or other type of virus or condition. If you throw up every time you take your medication, talk to your rheumatologist about other options for treating your RA. The goal of the meds is to enhance your life, not make you miserable in another way.

19
Gas

"I feel as bloated as the Goodyear blimp."

It was a balmy summer's evening not too long after I started the TNF blocker Enbrel. I'd been out for dinner with friends, enjoying tiger shrimp sautéed in lots of garlic. Meandering down the street towards home, replete with good food and good company, we chatted about this, that and the other thing. As I opened my mouth to reply to a question, a surprise belch escaped my body, and when I say "belch," I don't mean a ladylike burp, not even an unladylike burp. No, I mean a belch of Olympic proportions, so loud I'm quite sure it rattled windows. The people waiting at the crosswalk a good fifteen yards ahead of me turned around in astonishment.

I tried to look innocent.

RA meds are famous for their gastrointestinal side effects and the biologics are particularly efficient in this, having the potential for making you as windy as a January day in Chicago. And when they hit you hard, it's the kind of wind that — especially in the beginning — cannot always be controlled. This means that in no time, you can become much less uptight about bodily functions. Hopefully, so will those around you.

Does that sound mortifying? It doesn't have to be. There are tricks to managing the gas that can keep it down to a dull roar or at least minimize it during occasions that shouldn't be accompanied by toots and burps.

Stay away from farty foods if you have to be around other people. Beans are famous for giving you gas, but there are a number of other foods and drinks that can make it hard to keep air from escaping. You might call them performance-enhancing drugs. These include garlic, spicy foods, anything deep-fried, milk and dairy products, soy, vegetables like cabbage, broccoli and cauliflower, bran, artificial sweeteners and drinks with bubbles like soda and beer. You likely already know what foods make you bloat, but you may find that once you're on RA meds, other foods get added to the list. Keeping a symptom diary will help you identify them (see Chapter 1).

Stock up on Gas-X and Beano. There are two types of over-the-counter medication that can help you. Beano contains an enzyme that helps prevent gas before it occurs. It should be taken with the food you know gives you gas.[64] Gas-X helps reduce and disperse trapped gas bubbles.[65] One may help you more than the other. As with all types of medication, how much they help can depend on the person. Ask your doctor or pharmacist for advice and try both to find out how they work for you.

Drink tea. There are a number of herbal teas that can be helpful in reducing gas. Stock up on peppermint, ginger and fennel teas and test all of them to find out what's most helpful. For some, drinking herbal teas throughout the day will be helpful, while others might prefer to only drink herbal teas when they feel particularly gassy. As mentioned in Chapter 18, peppermint and ginger teas can also be helpful in dealing with nausea.

As your body gets used to the medication, the gas will most likely simmer down. You might still get bloated and gassy, especially for the first few days after you take your meds, but not in the same way you may have experienced in the beginning. After a few months, I no longer belched loud enough to make the windows rattle. Your body will also adapt to certain foods. For instance, eating high fiber foods is not only good for your body, but can also help you manage the constipation that sometimes accompanies RA meds (see Chapter 20). Although increasing your fiber intake can also make you gassier at first, your body will get used to the higher amount of fiber, and the gas will decrease again.

Managing gas becomes second nature the same way as managing other side effects does: it becomes a regular part of your routine. You'll learn when you can indulge in a meal of chili with garlic bread and when you should eat a less wind-inducing diet. Knowing what can help reduce the gas can make it even more manageable. Keep in mind, though, gas is a natural byproduct of eating. We all burp and fart. In fact, some intrepid researcher discovered that on average, human beings fart fourteen times a day. RA meds may increase that number, but with a combination of watching what you eat, over-the-counter meds and a relaxed attitude, it won't interfere with your life.

20
Constipation and Diarrhea

"Someone put a cork in me and I haven't gone for days!"

Moving below the belly button in our top to bottom journey of possible side effects, gas isn't the only byproduct of RA meds and various painkillers. These drugs can also influence your bowel movements, causing either diarrhea or, more frequently, constipation. As with nausea and high levels of acid in your stomach, one of the first tools you can use is acidophilus, a probiotic. It helps to regulate and normalize the bacteria in your gut, which can ease both constipation and diarrhea. Start slow, with one dose a day with a meal, and if that works well, try two doses a day. As I mentioned in Chapter 18, if the acidophilus makes your bowel movements a bit too loose, reducing the dose usually resolves the issue.

The best way to manage constipation is to increase the amount of fiber you consume. You can do this by increasing the fiber in your diet or with one of the many fiber supplements available in the pharmacy area of your supermarket. Remember to drink lots and lots of water at the same time — fiber needs water to work its magic. Too little water and you might become even more constipated.

Personally, I'm a big fan of incorporating fiber in my diet. There are so many delicious foods that are high in fiber. By changing your diet to one that is healthier, you're helping your body be as strong as possible. What works well can vary from person to person, so play around until you discover what is best for you. Some suggestions are:

Breakfast

The high fiber cereals tend to be along the top shelves at the supermarket, whereas the sugary, refined cereals that aren't good for you inhabit the lower shelves. Look up and check for Bran Flakes, All-Bran, All-Bran Buds, Shreddies and many others. Muesli is a very tasty mix of oat flakes, various grains, dried fruits and nuts and can be a terrific way to start the day. Eat it hot or cold with milk or yogurt. Check the label — some brands of muesli don't have as much fiber as you might need. You can also look up recipes on the Internet and make your own. And of course, there are oats. Starting the day with a helping of oatmeal gives you a good foundation. It's very filling, which means you're less likely to snack on pastries throughout the morning. Oatmeal can also help lower your cholesterol.

Some people shy away from All-Bran with milk because they think it tastes like soggy cardboard. Try sprinkling a handful on yogurt where it can stay crunchy, offering a nice contrast and texture to the creamy dairy product. Yogurt is also a natural source of probiotic, which can help your gastrointestinal system stay healthier.

Lunch and Dinner

Instead of refined white sandwich bread in plastic bags, look for grainy bread in the bakery. Luckily, it's much easier to find really good bread now than it was in the past. If you can't quite get used to the crunch, the softer breads that come in plastic bags also have a variety of higher grain options.

For sandwiches, try hummus as a spread instead of mayonnaise. Hummus is a dip made from chickpeas, tahini (sesame seed paste) and olive oil, and it comes in many delicious flavors.

White rice can make you more constipated, so try brown rice or wild rice blends instead. When pasta is on the menu, buy whole grain pasta instead of the more standard option.

Beans of all kinds are excellent sources of fiber and can easily be included in meals. They can be used in hot dishes like chili, soups or side dishes or cold in different types of salads.

You can also include fresh fruits and vegetables with your lunch or dinner. If you steam veggies, don't overdo it — steam them for only a few minutes. This will leave a bit of a crunch, as well as keeping the good stuff like vitamins and fiber intact.

Snacks

Snacks can be healthy and taste good, too. In between meals, graze on healthy, high fiber snacks like dry Bran Flakes (trust me — quite delicious, especially if you mix them with raisins), granola and trail mix. Fruit can also help get things going, especially fruit with pits such as plums, cherries and peaches. Dried versions of these fruits, including prunes, can be very effective, as well. You can start your morning with some stewed prunes, which can taste very nice. Stew a larger portion, keep it in the fridge and eat a bit of it with cold milk. I grew up in Denmark and it's an actual dessert there — a very yummy one, too. As well, one of the reasons that an apple a day keeps the doctor away is because apples can help keep you regular. Be sure to leave the skin on — it's where most of the fiber is.

Other

Adding more fiber to your diet is not the only way of solving constipation. The supplement bromelain is an enzyme extracted from pineapple. It has a couple of different uses and can be very helpful in moving along your bowels. To aid with digestion, take it with food. As mentioned in Chapter 14, bromelain can also work as a bit of an anti-inflammatory. To use it for that purpose, it should be taken a couple of hours away from food.

If you've ever eaten too many Licorice Allsorts, you know what black licorice can do for constipation. Although some people paradoxically get more constipated when eating licorice, most people react the other way. Keep in mind that licorice contains sugar, so use in moderation to avoid cavities and weight gain. Black licorice may raise your blood pressure, so go easy if you have hypertension.

There may be times when fiber alone won't do the trick. This may be especially true if you're taking narcotic painkillers (opioids) that can also cause constipation. In such cases, speak to your doctor about additional help like stool softeners. Such medications should usually only be taken temporarily, so if your constipation is persistent despite your efforts, discuss solutions with your doctor or pharmacist.

Diarrhea

Some of the RA meds can cause loose stool or diarrhea, either temporarily for a few days following taking your medication or on a more chronic basis. As with most meds, some people tolerate a particular medication very well, whereas others end up frequently running for the washroom. This can continue for several weeks, sometimes even after stopping the medication.

If things are bad and include frequent trips to the washroom as well as nausea, a tip you may remember from childhood to deal with the stomach flu can be helpful. Go on the BRAT diet: Bananas, Rice (white), Applesauce and Toast until you're better. Go back and read Chapter 18 again for tips on how to manage the nausea. You can also incorporate some bland foods such as steamed fish and chicken, to make sure you get adequate protein.

If things get really bad, it may help to use a symptom diary for a few weeks (see Chapter 1) to help identify what helps and what makes it worse. Over-the-counter medications such as Gravol and Imodium can help ease stomach upset and stop the diarrhea. However, if you find that your diarrhea is long-lasting, unmanageable, weakens you or limits your ability to lead your life, talk to your doctor about other treatment options for your RA.

If your problem is temporary (only lasting a couple of days), changing your diet to include foods that are constipating may help control the diarrhea. Foods that may cause constipation include blueberries, salted snacks, beef, nuts and sugar. You can also add acidophilus or another probiotic to your daily routine, as it can be helpful to manage both constipation and diarrhea. This regulates the bacteria in your gut and can therefore help keep your digestive system's response to medication from getting too extreme.

Whether your issue is constipation or diarrhea, time and trying different foods will tell you what works for you and what doesn't. For instance, if you know which kinds of foods make you fart, you may know what can ease constipation — farting can be one of the first signs that your bowels are getting ready to move. On the other hand, foods that make you fart, such as beans and other high fiber foods, will usually make diarrhea worse. Your body will have its own special needs. Paying attention to what you eat and listening to your body will help you know what those are.

These last three chapters were sort of a mini section on their own within the larger discussion of side effects. RA meds are well-known for messing with the gastrointestinal system, so chances are you'll refer to these chapters more than the rest. The good news is that these kinds of side effects can usually be managed with some common sense tricks, many of which happen to taste good, too. Sometimes, RA meds give you the opportunity to discover new and wonderful things about the world. For me, that discovery was roasted garlic hummus and best of all, I get to claim that it's medicinal! I hope you will be able to make your own culinary discovery.

21
Dryness, Thirst and Skin Care

"I'm so dry, I'm dusty."

A sense of decorum was the only thing that kept me from permanently attaching my mouth to the kitchen faucet and turning on the cold water. I was so thirsty — thirstier than I'd ever been in my life. I felt like the desert under the hot noonday sun where every splash of water is instantly absorbed, leaving no trace on the dry, dusty ground.

I hadn't been on Enbrel, one of the biologic medications, for very long before the dryness began. It started with the endless thirst, then moved onto my skin and my eyes became dry, as well. I eventually switched to Humira, another biologic, but the dryness stuck around.

The good news is that if you experience this kind of side effect, it's usually one that's just annoying.

The thirst takes some getting used to, but the solution is simple: just drink when you need it. Make sure you choose something that's actually hydrating and doesn't have a high sugar content — carbonated pop won't do much to quench your thirst. As well, anything caffeinated has a tendency to make you thirstier, so water and juice are better choices. Keep the juice to reasonable quantities — remember, it has sugar, too — and if you battle sinus-related side effects, make some of it 100% pineapple juice (see Chapter 14). You can try some hot water with a small slice of lemon and/or ginger — it's refreshing and can help keep your stomach calm (see Chapter 18).

If you've reached your limit on how much water you can drink before you start sloshing when you move, or you're in a situation where you won't be able to go to the bathroom for several hours, other tricks can be helpful. Suck on mints or chew gum, but consider buying the sugar-free options to prevent cavities. Sucking on a small piece of lemon can also get your salivary glands going so you don't feel quite as thirsty anymore. As a last resort, my doctor once told me that if you don't drink for about an hour, the feeling of being thirsty goes away. I've tried it and found she was right. However, use that trick only when you absolutely have to — thirst is your body's signal that it needs liquid. Ignoring that urge too much can make you dehydrated.

Dry Mouth

Thirst can be a symptom of dry mouth, a potential side effect of medication. It can also be related to other health conditions, such as nasal allergies that make you a "mouth breather," or it can be a possible symptom of Sjögren's (pronounced SHOW-grins) Syndrome. Some people with RA develop Sjögren's, an autoimmune disorder that affects the mucous membranes and glands that produce moisture. That means the first symptoms of Sjögren's are usually dry mouth and dry eyes.[66] This is another moment when it's a good idea to breathe deeply and not assume the worst. If you notice these kinds of symptoms after you start your medication, they are probably a side effect, not another autoimmune disease.

Regardless of the cause, dry mouth can be very uncomfortable. We need saliva to keep our mouths clean and moist and to digest our food. Saliva also protects your teeth and gums from bacteria that can cause cavities and gingivitis (inflammation of the gums). If your mouth is very dry, you may have a higher risk of developing cavities and gum disease.[67]

Drinking water and chewing gum help, but sometimes not enough. Involve your dentist in your care. Dentists specialize in the health of the mouth and are well qualified to deal with issues pertaining to this area of your body. As well, they're more likely to know of products that can treat conditions that involve your mouth. For instance, my dental hygienist told me about a product called Biotene, which helps relieve symptoms of mild to severe dry mouth. Biotene comes in a number of different forms, including a rinse, spray, toothpaste, gum and gel.

Taking Care of Your Eyes

Some people find that the dryness moves on to other parts of their bodies, too. One of the first places you may notice this is in your eyes. If they burn and feel dry, speak to your doctor. It's important to stay ahead of dry eyes — inadequate lubrication can cause damage to your cornea, which can be quite painful and will take a while to heal. Most likely this problem can be managed with over-the-counter saline eye drops three to four times a day. However, if you have significant symptoms of dryness, especially in your mouth and eyes, talk to your doctor about a referral to an ophthalmologist or optometrist. The best person to take care of your eyes is someone who specializes in that part of the body.

Getting your eyes checked every year is usually a good idea when you have RA. Not only will you find out if you need glasses so you can see clearly, but you'll also be doing your best to take care of your eyes. If you develop any problems, there's a greater likelihood of catching them early.

Skin Care

If the dryness affects your skin, find a good moisturizer. You may have to try several different body lotions before you find one that can see you through the day. For me, that moisturizer is Aveeno, but something else may work better for you. If necessary, use the lotion in both the morning and evening. Shea butter and coconut oil are also terrific moisturizers — your local health food store will probably carry them.

You may also want to consider giving up scented soap and shower gel, as they can dry out your skin. In my experience, fragrance-free goat's milk soap can change your hands from being terribly dry with cracked skin to being soft again. And these days, goat's milk soap doesn't smell like a barnyard at all!

Some people's hands get so dry that they experience cracks at the tips of their fingers, particularly in winter. It seems to happen especially to people who wash their hands frequently, such as healthcare providers, mechanics or parents. And that's before you add RA and medications that dry you out! If your fingers start cracking, there are a number of different creams and lotions that can heal the cracks.

Aquaphor is one of the best healers I've ever tried. Your pharmacist may be able to special order it, but it is also available online. Tea tree oil may also heal the cracks. Since this kind of extreme dryness often happens to mechanics, specialist hardware stores sometimes stock a cream that can help. The absolute best for cracked hands is Bag Balm, a cream used for cracked udders on cows. It's sold for people too, as more and more are discovering just how good it is for healing your hands. An Internet search will help you find places where you can buy it.

Women may also experience vaginal dryness. This topic is covered in Chapter 23.

Rashes, Skin Hardening and Photosensitivity

Rashes can also be a side effect of some of the RA meds, especially drugs like the TNF blocker Enbrel. Most of the time, these rashes are an irritant that can be managed. One of the common side effects of injectable biologics is a skin reaction at the site where you inject the meds. For most, that's as far as it goes. Switching injection sites every time you do your shot should take care of it. You may also want to discuss this with your doctor for more tips on how to manage this kind of reaction.

Some people may experience rashes on other parts of their bodies. This happened to me when I was on Enbrel, and they seemed to be related to my skin getting incredibly sensitive. Most of my rashes appeared in areas where my clothes rubbed against my skin. They were terribly itchy, like the worst mosquito bite I've ever had. This caused me to come up with the word "skingasm" to describe the intense relief of scratching really hard.

There are a few types of rashes that may indicate a rare but severe side effect. A severe rash could mean that you're having an extreme reaction to the medication and need to contact your doctor. As is always the case with a serious reaction to any medication, if you experience difficulty breathing, call 911.

If you develop a butterfly-shaped rash across your nose and cheeks, it may be an indication of another serious side effect. Although rare, one of the side effects of Enbrel is lupus, an autoimmune disease that attacks tissue and organs. The butterfly rash is a classic symptom of lupus, so if you develop this, contact your doctor as soon as possible. If you do get lupus as a side effect of a TNF blocker, it may disappear again when the medication is stopped.

If you get benign rashes as a side effect, it is very possible to find a way to reduce the itch. It is also possible to learn to largely ignore it. I have very limited mobility and often can't reach an itchy place, forcing me to get very acquainted with my willpower. This has taught me that if you wait a while, the itch tends to go away. Learning to ignore the itch is a good idea not just because it means you can focus on other things, but also because scratching constantly can cause patches of thick, hardened skin. This is called lichenification and looks and feels sort of like a callus.[68]

There are also some reports of Enbrel causing skin hardening without the scratching. Mostly, this seems to happen as a reaction to your injection when a small, hard lump forms under the skin at the injection site. Usually, it disappears after a few days. Alternating injection sites between different areas of your stomach or thighs can help reduce this reaction.

For me, the benefits of being on Enbrel still vastly outweighed the itching and redness from the rashes. My dermatologist gave me a steroid cream, but in the end, I found Bach Rescue Remedy cream to be more effective in dealing with the problem. Rescue Remedy is a combination of several different flower extracts and is available in health food stores. In its liquid form, it can be very effective in helping you to calm down when you're anxious or upset (see Chapter 13). Rescue Remedy cream can work wonders to calm irritated nerves in your skin so the itching stops. Calendula cream, containing the medicinal variety of the pot marigold plant, can also be very helpful. It can also be found in health food stores.

Certain RA medications, such as Plaquenil and some of the biologics, may also cause photosensitivity, meaning you get very sensitive to the rays of the sun. Add to this the fact that some TNF blockers (Enbrel, Humira) lead to a slightly increased risk of developing skin cancer, and familiarizing yourself with sunscreen and sunblock becomes a must. Pick a product that has broad-spectrum UVA and UVB protection and an SPF level of at least thirty. Remember that sunscreen offers added protection from the sun, but doesn't completely block it. Baking for hours at the beach is not a good idea — instead, use a snazzy hat, cover up and stay in the shade. You should also keep an eye on your skin to make sure you catch new moles quickly. Getting checked by a dermatologist for suspicious moles once a year is an important part of preventive healthcare for everyone and especially for people who are on certain RA meds.

As you come to the end of this chapter, remember that dry mouth, skin and eyes, rashes and sun irritation happen all the time to everyone. It most likely has happened to you at different times throughout your life before you started RA meds. This means that a patch of dry or red, irritated skin is probably nothing to worry about. If your eyes are dry and burn, you may have seasonal allergies. If you're itchy, it could be just one of those things. The key is to remember that a persistent symptom that gets worse after you take your medication may be a side effect. If the problem is not severe, pull out your trusty symptom diary (see Chapter 1) and keep an eye on things for a couple of weeks. Then bring it up the next time you see your rheumatologist or family doctor.

22
Bladder

"Why do I have to pee all the time?"

Most of us have known this feeling. You have an awareness of your bladder that ranges from noticing it's there to a sort of dull ache, and you have to pee if you as much as look at a glass of water. When you do go to the bathroom, it burns or you feel as if you can't quite finish. Which can only mean one thing, right? Call it urinary tract infection (UTI), bladder infection or cystitis — an infection by any other name still stings when you pee.

Just as you may be more vulnerable to sinus infections if you are on medication that suppresses your immune system, you may also be more at risk for bladder infections. Women tend to be more prone to UTIs because everything is so close together in their genital area, but men get them, too.

Although you may be more vulnerable to UTIs, you can reduce the risk by taking good care of your bladder. Having fewer bladder infections will not only make you more comfortable, but will also reduce the amount of antibiotics you take.

Drink cranberry juice. Research has indicated that cranberry juice can prevent bacteria from turning into a bladder infection. Ingredients in the cranberry juice prevent *E. coli* bacteria from sticking to other bacteria, thereby limiting its ability to grow.[69] According to the studies, cranberry cocktail will do the trick, but several health professionals (including my naturopath and a nurse practitioner) have told me that real cranberry juice without added sugar can be more effective. If you choose to go this route, look for the brand names R.W. Knudsen Family or Black River in your supermarket or health food store.

The no sugar added kind of cranberry juice comes in a concentrate that you can drink once a day. You should be aware that it can be pretty sour, so don't try to savor it. Hold your nose and gulp down a shot of it. If the taste is too much for you, mixing it with water and adding some ice dilutes the sourness and makes a refreshing drink. You can also take cranberry capsules if the taste of the juice doesn't appeal to you or if it aggravates the acid in your stomach. However, my naturopath also told me that drinking the juice is more effective than the capsules in helping you stay ahead of bladder infections.

You should also drink lots of fluids in general, especially water. The more you drink, the more you flush out your bladder, which keeps bacteria from accumulating. The less bacteria that gathers in your bladder, the lower the risk of infection and the better you feel.

In addition to drinking cranberry juice, there are a number of other simple actions that can help reduce the risk of bladder infections.

Use the washroom as frequently as you need it and try to avoid holding your urine for long periods of time. If you're a woman, wipe from front to back after you pee or have a bowel movement. This prevents transferring bacteria from your rectal area to the opening of your urethra where the urine comes out.

It's also a good idea for women to pee after sex, as this can flush out bacteria that may have been pushed inside the urethra during intercourse. You may also want to wash after sex to remove bacteria. And while we are on the topic of washing, avoid bubble baths — they may feel wonderful, but they can irritate the genital area. Take showers or baths without the bubbles.

Both men and women should keep their genital area clean and dry. Cotton underwear is your friend, as this material absorbs moisture and helps keep you dry. Other types of fabric that include synthetic materials such as nylon do not absorb moisture and can therefore create an environment where bacteria can thrive.

If you have symptoms of a bladder infection, such as needing to pee often, feelings of urgency and burning or stinging when you use the washroom, see a doctor to get tested. Don't try to wait it out — if you have a UTI, waiting will just make it worse. If you need antibiotics, take them and drink a lot of water. You may also want to increase the amount of cranberry juice you drink.

Some people who are on a biologic drug may experience symptoms of a UTI without actually having an infection. This can happen especially for a couple of days right after taking the medication. I'm one of the "lucky" ones in that respect. For a long time I thought I had frequent bladder infections, but the tests were all negative. Eventually, I figured out the link between my shot and the symptoms. After I get my injection, I spend a couple of days having muscle pains all over my body that feel like a sort of light muscle cramping. Since the bladder is a muscle, mine does some spasming, as well, and I visit the washroom a bit more often. If you experience this kind of side effect, rest assured it can be managed fairly easily.

Over the years, I've learned to live with these symptoms to the point where I hardly notice them anymore. My main coping technique is to pay attention to the timing of drinking liquids. For instance, I stop drinking about two hours before going to bed. If I don't, I have to get up in the middle of the night to visit the washroom. As I need assistance to get out of bed and onto the toilet, getting up at 3 a.m. to pee can be difficult. Many people with RA also find that a good night's uninterrupted sleep helps their pain levels. If this is you, try paying attention to how long it takes for a glass of water to pass through you.

If your bladder spasms, it can make it difficult to empty it. Staying on the toilet for an extra few minutes can be very helpful. Don't rush it, don't strain and be patient — you'll be surprised how much is left in your bladder even though you thought you were done.

If you experience this side effect and the spasms lead to losing a few drips of urine every now and again, don't worry — you'll share the symptom with pretty much any woman who has ever given birth. You can buy pads and pantyliners made specifically for this purpose in drug stores and supermarkets.

Doing Kegel exercises several times a day may help to strengthen and relax the bladder muscles for both men and women.[70] Strengthening the bladder in this way can help control symptoms of occasional leaking of urine and may also circumvent the spasms. Sometimes, if you tighten and release a muscle, it can make the spasms stop. In this type of exercise, you tighten the muscles of the pelvic floor like you would if you were trying to stop peeing in midstream. The great thing about these exercises is that they can be done anywhere — waiting for a red light to turn green, in an elevator, while you cook dinner or sitting at your desk. Talk to your family doctor to get more information on how to do Kegel exercises correctly.

If your bladder spasms change from manageable to having a significant impact on your quality of life, it may be time to talk to your doctor. If you are uncomfortable, spend too much time in the bathroom or experience higher and more frequent pain levels in your bladder, you may benefit from medications that can help relax and minimize bladder spasms. If you see a doctor of naturopathic medicine, they may also be able to help you with either acupuncture or homeopathic remedies, such as Arnica for pain or APIS 30 for burning. Keep in mind that homeopathic and natural medicine is still medicine. Don't try to medicate yourself — consult an expert, such as a naturopath, to make sure that any such treatment doesn't interfere with medication you're already taking.

Keep an eye on what's happening down below. If you experience side effects such as bladder spasms, pain or frequent UTIs that limit you as much as active RA, it may be time to talk to your rheumatologist about looking into other types of treatment.

People's individual experiences with bladder-related symptoms are just that: individual. Most never experience any symptoms beyond an occasional UTI that they might've had anyway, while some, like me, learn to live with a new awareness of that area of their anatomy. If you end up joining this particular club — shall we call ourselves Bladder Spasmers, Inc? — most of the time, it's a manageable symptom. As with other side effects, you learn to take inventory of the impact on your life of occasional, usually temporary symptoms and the odd UTI versus the impact of active RA. It's all about perspective.

23

Hormones, Sex Drive and Other Unmentionables

"Where did my libido go?"

And now we come to the chapter that might make you squirm a little. It's one thing to discuss side effects related to an acidic stomach, gas or your blood pressure, but sex? Genital health? This is the point when many of us start cringing and that seems to include the field of medicine.

Both medications and RA itself can lead to problems related to genital health and function. There isn't much talk of this and not much research either — the medical profession doesn't tend to look too closely at sexual health or even side effects related to your nether bits. Sometimes, I wonder if they're shy or just being deliberately obtuse.

Ignoring this topic does no one any favors. It leaves people with RA isolated and without recourse to deal with issues related to sexual and genital health. It leaves doctors ignorant of the true impact of RA and medications. Although many of these types of side effects tend to be relatively rare, being aware that they may happen will help you deal with the situation if it does. Talking openly to your doctor about sexuality and your genital health will help you and may also help to create awareness of these issues within the medical profession. This can help other people with RA in the future.

Let's take a deep breath, gird our loins (!) and talk about it.

Women

One of the reasons you're more prone to developing sinus infections if you're on a biologic medication seems, in my experience, to be related to an increased production of mucus in the sinus cavity. Other areas of your body also produce mucus, including your vaginal area. You may therefore experience some vaginal discharge for a few days after taking your medication. It usually looks like the clear discharge you can get around the time of ovulation. As long as it remains clear and odorless, you should be OK.

Some women report more frequent yeast infections when taking immunosuppressant medications like methotrexate and the biologics. If you experience discharge that is not clear, smells off or if your vaginal area itches, it may be an infection. If you have these kinds of symptoms, don't be shy. Make an appointment to see your family doctor to get checked. As with most infections, the sooner you deal with it, the easier it will be to treat.

RA meds can also have an impact on your menstrual cycle, although it's hard to predict which way it's going to go. Depending on the drug and how you react to it, your periods can get heavier or lighter, more irregular or as regular as clockwork and your PMS can get worse or easier. The bottom line is this: if you notice a change in your periods that concerns you, talk to your doctor.

Several of the RA meds can cause dryness, not just in the eyes and mouth, but the vagina, as well. As estrogen levels decrease with the onset of menopause, this can become more pronounced. Between 10% and 40% of postmenopausal women experience shrinking, thinning and a decrease in muscle mass of the tissue in the vagina. The medical name for this condition is atrophic vaginitis — awful name, isn't it? It can cause irritation, itching, dryness and pain during intercourse.[71]

Vaginal dryness at any age can often be managed by using plenty of lubrication during intercourse, such as K-Y Jelly or Astroglide. Remember that your lubricant should be water-based. Petroleum-based lubricant, such as Vaseline, can break down condoms. As well, if you're in a monogamous relationship and not using condoms, petroleum-based lubricants can introduce bacteria into the body and increase your risk of infection.

Increasing blood circulation to the vagina can help keep that area healthy, potentially reducing the symptoms of dryness and thinning of the vaginal wall. The easiest way to increase blood circulation is to have frequent sex and/or masturbate more often.[72] This may be one of the most fun medical recommendations I've ever heard!

If you have vaginal dryness, don't assume you have conditions with terrible names. However, if your symptoms are persistent, difficult to manage and impact your sex life, make an appointment with your doctor to talk about it. They may be able to give you more insight into what's going on, as well as suggestions on how to deal with the situation. You may also want to talk to them about a prescription for estrogen cream — it can be very helpful in managing these types of symptoms.[73]

Medications for RA can impact a woman's sex drive, although — big surprise — there doesn't seem to be much research on the topic. Your sex drive can also be affected by hormonal changes as you age, as well as psychological and emotional factors (more on this topic below). If you're experiencing a decrease in your sex drive that is unusual, see your doctor. Applying a progesterone cream may be helpful in increasing libido for some women, especially if the changes in sex drive are related to hormonal changes. Your family doctor or OB/GYN will be able to give you more information about this option.

Because of the lack of studies on women's libido, it may be more of a challenge to find something that can help you. Go to a women's bookstore, find a sex shop run or staffed by women or look around on the Internet, particularly in forums where you can talk to other women who have experienced problems with a low sex drive. They will be able to share their experiences and tips on how to manage. Finding out what works for you might take a while. Don't rush it, approach it with patience and a sense of humor and remember that there's more to you than your sexuality.

Men

There's a pretty good understanding that women's libido is affected by a number of factors and may wax and wane. Men, on the other hand, seem to be assumed to be robots, expected to be able to spring to attention (if you'll forgive the phrase) at all times. It's not like that. Men, too, have changes in desire. Most men — those with RA and those without — will at some point in their lives experience technical difficulties in the erection department. Usually this is temporary and occurs at times of stress or fatigue (more on this topic below). However, other factors such as age, medications or other medical conditions may affect your erections in a more significant way. If you frequently have trouble getting or keeping an erection, you may have erectile dysfunction (ED). For men who live with RA, there are two general causes of ED.

If you've been having RA flares for a long time, it can affect the function of your testicles, causing a condition called hypogonadism.[74] Essentially, it's low levels of testosterone and it can cause symptoms like erectile dysfunction, fatigue, decreased sex drive, depression, anxiety, hot flashes, frequent urination and gynecomastia (breast enlargement). The second cause of ED in men with RA is medication. Certain drugs — for instance methotrexate — may impact your sexual health and affect your ability to get an erection.

If you've noticed changes in your sex drive or other symptoms like the ones listed above, ask your doctor to test your testosterone levels. It's a simple blood test that indicates whether your ability to produce testosterone has been affected. If your levels are low, you can be treated with testosterone replacement therapy. ED can also be treated with medication like Viagra and Cialis, penile injections (I can see you wincing now) and devices such as vacuum cylinders and penile implants. Some of those treatments sound quite terrifying. The point is that there are ways of managing this condition and some are as un-scary as taking a pill.

If you do have problems achieving an erection, have an open and honest discussion with your doctor. You may also want to do some online research and find information and tips in forums where men with ED share their experiences. Make sure you research any suggested treatment thoroughly, and check with your doctor before taking anything recommended by someone on the Internet. As is so often the case, if it sounds too good to be true, it probably is — particularly if it's a late-night infomercial or unsolicited email.

Staying Safe when You Have Sex

For some people with RA, safe sex is about more than protecting themselves against sexually transmitted diseases. Two medications used for RA can cause severe birth defects (see Chapter 27). If you are on methotrexate or Arava, it is very, very important that you use birth control that has a high rate of success in preventing pregnancy. In fact, it's probably not a bad idea to double up on birth control methods, using for instance, a combination of an intrauterine device (IUD) and condom or birth control pills and condoms or another combination. This isn't just important for women to remember. As of yet, there isn't any specific evidence that Arava can be passed through semen and cause birth defects, but researchers have recommended that men be extremely careful nonetheless.[75] You don't want to take any chances with this one.

This potentially serious side effect is another reason you should be honest with your doctor about your sexual health. Although your RA may affect your sex life — and more on that in a minute — for most of us, our diagnosis doesn't come with an automatic entry into celibacy. Doctors are human and prone to their own biases. That means that some doctors assume that a chronic illness is incompatible with a healthy sex life. Make sure you mention that you are sexually active when you get a prescription for a new medication. This will help you and your doctor start a discussion about how to stay safe.

More About Sex and Libido

For both men and women, sex drive isn't just related to specific physiological responses caused by RA or side effects from medication. Although technically outside the scope of the chapter on side effects of medication, I have a feeling a lot of you have more questions about sex with RA, so please allow me a brief sidetrack.

Libido is a complicated phenomenon, affected by physiological events in the body, as well as psychological and emotional responses to what's going on in your life. If you're feeling crappy because you're flaring, sex is probably not going to be foremost in your mind. If you're hurting, you may be afraid that sex will make it worse, so you put it on the shelf for a while. If you're having a hard time adjusting to RA and it's messing with your self-esteem and body image, it can be hard to feel sexy. All of these situations and many more can have an effect on your libido.

And it's completely normal. In fact, it happens to everyone, with or without a chronic illness. Stress, anxiety, depression and intense focus on other things have a tendency to shove sex to the bottom of the priority list. No one is ready to go at a moment's notice, 24/7.

If you experience a low sex drive and it bothers you, talk to your doctor to find out if there's a physiological reason. Also, don't forget that the most important people involved in issues related to your sex drive are you and your partner. Intimacy is an important part of relationships. Without it, partners can feel isolated from each other at a time when they most need to be connected. Keeping the lines of communication open is essential to help each of you understand what the other is feeling. Physical intimacy is also essential, but if one of you is having a really bad day and not up to sex, cuddling can go a long way towards filling that need.

Having RA doesn't mean the end of your sex life. In fact, there's no reason why you shouldn't have a very good time with your partner. RA does add the need for good communication, so both of you have a better understanding of the potential impact of fatigue and pain on what happens in the bedroom... or kitchen... or hallway (I'm not judgy). Keep talking, involve a counselor if necessary and keep loving each other.

24
Weight Changes

"My pants are too big. My shirt is too tight."

When I was thirteen, prednisone saved my life but also caused me to gain weight. A lot of weight. Thirty years later, when I was forty-three, Enbrel saved my life but also caused me to lose weight. A lot of weight.

One potential side effect of some RA medications can be changes in your weight. Although weight gain is the most common, some may also react by losing weight. Either way, the changes in your body can play havoc with your idea of who you are and your self-esteem.

We live in a culture that values being thin, especially for women. How thin is considered desirable varies. The ideal can be slim, yet healthy. It can also be the kind of thin that is only possible if you live on water and the odd leaf of lettuce while exercising six hours a day with a personal trainer. This is not healthy for anyone.

Men don't have it easy either. These days, the male ideal is to have a lot of muscles. As with being thin, achieving this level of muscle definition usually takes a personal trainer and a lot of time in the gym. Not realistic for most people who have jobs, kids and bills to pay.

The first step to find out if you should do something about your weight is to calculate your body mass index (BMI). BMI was developed by Adolphe Quetelet, a nineteenth century Belgian statistician. It is a measure of your weight in relation to your height that can be used to tell you whether you need to lose or gain weight.

To calculate BMI, use the following steps:[76]

Using metric measurements:
- Take your weight in kilograms (kg)
- Divide your weight by your height in meters (m)
- Divide the result again by your height in meters (m)
- The result is your BMI

For Imperial measurements:
- Take your weight in pounds (lb)
- Multiply your weight by 703
- Divide the result by your height in inches (in)
- Divide the result again by your height in inches (in)
- The result is your BMI

On the other hand, if you're like me and the idea of math makes your brain hurt, checking Google for the term "body mass index" will give you all sorts of links to sites that will calculate your BMI with no effort on your part. You can also speak to your doctor — chances are they have a poster about BMI in their office.

Regardless of how you find out what your BMI is, the number will tell you where you are in the range from underweight to overweight:[77]

- Below 18.5 – Underweight
- 18.5–24.9 – Normal
- 25–29.9 – Overweight
- 30 and above – Obese

If your BMI is below 25, you don't need to lose weight, no matter what the snarky voice in the mirror says. You may have a bit of bloat — cutting down on salt might take care of it — or need to tone your stomach muscles, but you are not as big as a house. It's quite all right to have a piece of chocolate or a nice meal with pasta and garlic bread without feeling guilty. Besides, in my opinion, guilt should never be applied to what we eat. It can lead to an unhealthy relationship with food, contributing to overeating or undereating. Moderation, on the other hand, is a much healthier concept when talking about food (and most other things in life).

If you fall into the overweight and above categories, losing weight will be good for you. Not because you'll look better — I firmly believe everyone is beautiful, no matter what they look like. It will, however, have a number of health benefits, such as reducing your risk of diabetes, heart disease and stroke. But that's not all. It will also be better for your joints. Extra pounds put extra stress on your joints, leading to an increase in pain and difficulty moving.

You've probably heard that fact before, and it can sound very theoretical, making it hard to apply to your everyday life. Putting your extra weight into another context can make it easier to see the impact it has on your body. Try putting twenty pounds worth of books, flour or fruit in a backpack. Put it on and carry it for half an hour or so, then take off the backpack again. How much lighter do you feel? Did you feel the relief in your joints when you put it down? Naturally, if you're having a really bad day or your RA is flaring, you might want to skip the Backpack Test — use your imagination instead.

Losing weight can be difficult when you have trouble moving because of RA, but it is possible.

First, to make sure your general health is good, book an appointment with your family doctor for a physical. If your cholesterol, blood pressure or blood sugar is up, you might want to ask for a referral to a dietitian or nutritionist who can help you rethink your approach to food. On the other hand, if you're only carrying a little bit of extra weight, don't stress yourself out. There are number of small changes you can use to lose weight in a healthy way and not feel like you're starving. If you need to lose more than a bit of weight, your doctor will be able to talk to you about options that can make the process more successful.

The first part of losing weight is to reduce calories. Cut down on junk food and sugary drinks (by the way, don't just do this if you need to lose weight — it's good for everyone's health). Reduce your portion sizes at meals, and don't have seconds unless you're hungry. If you feel full before you've eaten everything on your plate, leave the rest. Change your snacks to healthy ones, such as fruit, vegetables and trail mix.

The second factor in losing weight is to use more calories. Try to move a bit more, even if it's only five minutes a day in the beginning. Doing chores around the house can count as being active — vacuuming the living room means you're moving. On bad days, even making lunch or a cup of tea counts as moving. Talk to your doctor about a referral to a physical therapist, who can help you put together an exercise program that will be safe for your joints (see Chapter 39).

If you're trying to lose weight, staying focused on small, attainable goals can make the process less overwhelming. Remember that losing just one pound takes four pounds of stress off your knees.[78] Every pound you lose is a victory in itself. Take it slow, gradually incorporating changes in your lifestyle that will help you be healthier. And don't forget to focus on enjoying your life as much as possible. That includes occasionally having a piece of cake or some popcorn with a good movie. As long as you have your doctor's blessing, laughing every day is more important than counting calories.

But what if you're underweight? A bit on the thin side is probably OK — again, check with your doctor to make sure that you are generally healthy. However, if the skin by your armpits is too loose or your head seems too big for your frame, you may have reached the point where people start wondering if you're anorexic. Enbrel made me lose so much weight that after being on it for a year, I had no belly fat left at all. Even extremely fit female athletes have some belly fat — it's simply how women are built. I was much too thin and needed to find ways to be and look healthier. If you're in a similar situation, ask your doctor for a referral to a nutritionist or dietitian who can help you find healthy ways to gain weight.

My nutritionist taught me a lot about how to increase calories in a good way. When told to gain weight, some jump on the idea of junk food as a solution. However, fast food is bad for you in so many ways —too much salt, too much grease — and should only be eaten occasionally.

Better ways to increase calories are to increase your portion sizes at your regular meals and to have more healthy snacks. You'll also be among a small and select group of people who don't have to worry about carbs, so go ahead and increase these types of foods in your diet. This can include fruits, vegetables like potatoes and corn, whole grains (pasta and brown rice) and legumes such as chickpeas and kidney beans.

Adding more calories to your diet may mean adding food rich in healthy fats, such as salmon or nuts and seeds, either in their natural form or in cashew, almond or sunflower seed spreads. You can also supplement your diet with protein bars or nutritional drinks like Ensure and Boost. If you're really skinny and your cholesterol level will allow it, seek inspiration in Julia Child's cooking — it uses lots of butter. Watch the movie *Julie & Julia* to get inspired and then pick up Julia Child's cookbook *Mastering the Art of French Cooking* (and also possibly some antacids). Enjoy experimenting with delicious meals. In some ways, you can consider yourself lucky — while people all around you are conscious of their waistlines, you don't have to be!

Weight changes are a little like allergies — almost everyone has them at some point in their life. If your cousin, your best friend, your dad and the receptionist at work are all trying to lose weight, you have company in the challenge. How it happened and how you deal with it may be a bit different than someone who doesn't have RA, but no one needs to know that if you don't feel like sharing it. Dealing with the change, especially if it's weight gain, is more important for you, though. It will make your joints feel and function better, improving your quality of life. And that's what it's all about.

25

Osteoporosis

"Pass the milk."

Osteoporosis is a condition in which the amount of calcium and minerals in your bones decreases. This causes the bones to become more porous and brittle and therefore more prone to breaking. It is generally more common in women, especially those who are postmenopausal — approximately 70% of people with osteoporosis are female.[79] However, a number of factors related to having RA can increase the risk of developing osteoporosis for both men and women.

RA itself is a risk factor for osteoporosis. Regular steroid use is also a risk factor. Since many people with RA are prescribed prednisone, you may have a double whammy of risk. Many people who have RA also take proton-pump inhibitor drugs to deal with stomach-related side effects, such as acid reflux and GERD (see Chapter 18). Prolonged use of PPIs may also be a risk factor in developing osteoporosis, making for a potential triple whammy of risk.[80]

With all these whammies, is it inevitable that you will get osteoporosis?

Absolutely not. It's still a good idea to be vigilant about preventing this condition, though. Talk to your doctor about getting a bone density scan. This gives you a baseline that tells you how healthy your bones are now and helps you track potential changes in the future. Once you've done that, set about building strong bones.

The first step in preventing osteoporosis is to make sure your diet contains the recommended amount of calcium: two servings a day for men and women younger than fifty and three servings a day for those over fifty.[81] Obvious sources of calcium are dairy products, such as milk, yogurt and cheese, as well as calcium-fortified foods and drinks, such as orange juice. If you're lactose intolerant, lactose-free milk will give you the calcium you need. For people who have milk allergies or simply don't like the stuff, soy milk fortified with calcium will do the same. Certain foods also contain calcium — examples include tofu, kale (a dark green, leafy vegetable) and broccoli.

Given the increased risk of osteoporosis that comes with having RA, you may also want to have a chat with your doctor about taking calcium supplements.

There are two kinds of calcium supplements: calcium carbonate and calcium citrate. Calcium carbonate is more commonly available and depends on stomach acid for absorption. It therefore works best when taken with food.[82] However, it can be hard to digest for some, leading to side effects such as stomach upset. One solution to this problem can be to visit your local health food store to buy calcium in liquid form. Another option is to look for a calcium citrate supplement. This kind of calcium is easily digested and absorbed by the body whether it's taken with food or without. It may also be easier to tolerate for people who already have stomach problems. It's important to be aware that calcium citrate should not be taken with antacids that contain aluminum.[83] Read the labels and ask your doctor's advice about this issue.

To find out how much calcium a particular supplement has, check the label for the amount of "elemental" calcium. For instance, a 1,250 mg tablet might have 500 mg of elemental calcium. That means you get 500 mg of calcium, not 1,250.[84] While you are reading the label, also check the other ingredients, especially if you have allergies to seafood or shellfish. Some calcium supplements use coral or oyster (sometimes also referred to as "natural source").[85] If you have these types of allergies, check with a pharmacist about your options.

Your pharmacist or doctor can also be a good source of information regarding interactions between supplements and medications. Calcium supplements can interact with several medications. This includes (somewhat ironically) decreasing the absorption of bisphosphonates, a type of drug used to treat osteoporosis.[86]

While you are in the supplement aisle, you may also want to consider picking up some vitamin D. This vitamin is essential for processing calcium and building strong bones. The National Institutes of Health's Office of Dietary Supplements recommends 600 IU daily for everyone between the ages of one and seventy.[87] This is generally considered a very low estimate. Most doctors, naturopaths and other healthcare professionals will recommend 1,000 IU of vitamin D a day, or more if you are vitamin D deficient. Vitamin D has also been shown to play a significant role in managing pain, so increasing your dosage will be helpful on a couple of levels.

The second part of building strong bones is to use them, especially in weight-bearing exercises. Walking is one of the best ways to reduce your risk of thinning bones, but this can be difficult if your RA means you have trouble moving around. Any amount of walking is better than none, so just moving around your house doing chores definitely counts. If you can do a bit more than that, you're doing OK.

Walking in shallow water may also help your bones and can be easier for people who have a lot of pain. There is some debate about whether the buoyancy that makes exercising in water easier on your joints negates any benefit in terms of osteoporosis. However, an increasing number of medical professionals and physical therapists say that walking in thigh- to hip-deep water will give you some benefit.[88]

When you talk to your doctor about bone density scans, you may also want to talk to them about getting a referral to physical therapy. A physical therapist can help you develop an exercise program that is tailored specifically to your needs. This can help you stay mobile and fit while protecting your joints from undue stress, as well as help you build stronger bones (see Chapter 39).

A bone density scan may indicate that you have osteoporosis or osteopenia — lower than normal bone density, but not quite enough to qualify as osteoporosis. If your bone density scan indicates that you have either of these conditions, your doctor may recommend medication to slow bone loss or help you build new bone. There are a number of medications on the market that are used to treat osteopenia and osteoporosis. There are three classes of drugs:

Antiresorptives slow down the resorption of bone, i.e. slowing down bone loss.

Anabolics build new bone.

Biologics are a type of biologic drug that slows down the production of bone-removing cells, stopping bone loss before it occurs. There are not the same kinds of biologics that are used for RA.[89]

Providing detail about the pros and cons of these medications is beyond my expertise, but I can offer some general suggestions. As is the case with any medical condition or when considering any medication, doing research is always a good idea. Make sure you know as much as possible about your condition and the treatment options available. When you see your doctor, bring a list of questions related to issues like prognosis, the possible side effects of medications and lifestyle choices that may help you manage your condition.

Your joints need all the help they can get to stay healthy. Making sure that the bones connected to the joints are as strong as they can be is just common sense. Stronger bones will help you stay as mobile as possible, especially as you age. Being aware that as a person with RA you may have increased risk of developing osteopenia or osteoporosis will help you stay ahead of changes to your bones. Talking to your doctor early on about the risk factors can help you and your medical team develop a strategy to protect the health of your bones.

26

A Hodgepodge of Other Side Effects

"But what about...?"

So far, this part of the book has taken you on a journey of potential side effects, moving from your head and down along your body. This chapter discusses a handful of possible side effects that didn't easily fit into one of the other chapters. You could argue that hair loss and headaches (for instance) belonged at the beginning of this section, but they didn't really fit into a chapter on mood changes. Hence the hodgepodge chapter.

Hair Loss

I had been flaring for a while and it was clearly time to step up treatment. My rheumatologist suggested I try methotrexate and I went away to do research and think about it. I thought about the flare and what it was doing to my joints. I thought about the pain I was in. Then I thought about the fact that methotrexate is a kind of chemotherapy drug. Sure, when prescribed for RA, it's taken in minuscule doses compared to what people with cancer receive, but still... And then I looked at the side effects, saw *hair loss* and everything screeched to a stop.

For a couple of days I seriously considered incurring joint damage and living in severe pain because I couldn't deal with the possibility of losing my hair. In the end, I got a grip and filled my prescription for methotrexate. And the only side effect I had related to my hair was that it got a bit dry and curlier.

Some people who take methotrexate do experience hair loss, also called alopecia. Before you panic, please remember that this side effect is fairly rare. Hair loss can also be a potential — and again usually rare — side effect of several other RA medications, such as Arava and Plaquenil.[90] Most people who take these medications do not lose their hair.

Nonetheless, if you do experience this particular side effect, it can be really alarming to look down in the shower and see what looks like half your hair swirling down the drain. Rest assured that most hair loss connected to using methotrexate for RA is not dramatic to the point of balding and can be temporary. Talk to your doctor about taking folic acid — it can often deal with the problem. You may also want to talk to your doctor or naturopath about vitamin B12 shots, which can sometimes help nourish your hair.

If the hair loss gets more dramatic and is not helped by folic acid or other supplements, you have a decision to make. You can talk to your doctor about stopping the drug, which in most cases stops the hair loss. You should be aware that it's important not to stop methotrexate suddenly, as it can trigger a huge flare. If you do want to try another medication, you should reduce methotrexate very slowly over time. Talk to your doctor about how to do this safely.

On the other hand, if methotrexate is working well for you, you may want to think about whether the benefits are big enough to make the hair loss tolerable. What does this drug do for your joints, your health in general and your quality of life? Is it possible for you to get comfortable with hair loss? Can you wrap your head around living with hair extensions, wigs, scarves, hats or rocking the bald look?

Men may have an easier time with this one. These days, many men choose to shave their heads rather than show encroaching baldness, and some shave their heads as a fashion statement in general. It's seen as sexy. Women, however, face an entirely different perception — our culture's ideas of femininity and sex appeal are very connected to a woman's hair.

We all have different lines drawn in the sand about side effects we will not accept. For some, losing their hair very much represents that line. Others will find a way to get comfortable with it, satisfied with the benefits their joints experience from the medication. There is no right or wrong here, only what you decide you can live with. And only you can make that decision.

Headaches/Migraines

Headaches are a side effect that seems to be associated with pretty much every medication out there. RA drugs are no different and may cause headaches with varying degrees of severity. Sometimes it's as mild as the pressure of a temporary sinus headache after you take your medication (especially one of the biologics). Sometimes, it's the daily throbbing and nausea of a migraine that seems to go on forever. The milder variety can be managed with over-the-counter medication. More rarely, people may get headaches that can mess them up for weeks, sending them to the doctor, getting test after test before they figure out what's going on.

If you do get headaches, try to remember that as with many other types of side effects, they may decrease or even disappear as your body gets used to the medication. Giving yourself a couple of months to settle down physically after adding a new medication may be all you need. However, as with many other types of side effects, if the headaches are severe, call your doctor to discuss what's happening. Bad headaches can have a significant impact on your life, making everything harder and decreasing your quality of life. Your doctor will be able to help you with medication that can treat the headaches and migraines for the length of time you feel is a reasonable trial period. If you continue to have severe medication-related headaches, remember that the goal of RA meds is to help you have a better life, not trade one kind of pain for another.

Mouth Ulcers

Mouth ulcers or sores can happen when you take certain medications, especially methotrexate. They usually look like round white spots or blisters with red borders and are also called canker sores. They can be located on the inside of your lips, your palate or gums. Canker sores are quite common in the general population and are usually primarily a nuisance. They can be a bit painful and, depending on where in the mouth they are located, get irritated when your teeth rub up against them.

One of the best ways of dealing with mouth ulcers that appear as a side effect to RA medication is to take folic acid. One study found that people taking methotrexate for RA could decrease their incidence of mouth ulcers by up to 79% by taking folic acid.[91] Some doctors recommend taking 1 mg of folic acid once a day, while others suggest you take 5 mg once a week. Talk to your rheumatologist about which option is best for you. In addition to folic acid, yogurt or acidophilus may also help prevent mouth sores.[92]

If you get mouth ulcers, here are a couple of suggestions to help them heal faster. Try rinsing with salt water several times a day. Salt water is a good way to deal with many issues in your mouth, including mouth ulcers, healing irritated gums, keeping an extraction site clean after you've had a tooth pulled and canker sores. Mix warm-ish water with salt — approximately half a teaspoon in 8 ounces of water — and stir until the salt is dissolved. If you don't want to get obsessive about the measurements of salt and water, dip a finger into the water to taste it. The water should taste salty, but not so salty that it burns. Swish a mouthful around in your mouth and spit it out. Repeat a couple of times and don't rinse with regular water afterwards. If your mouth ulcers are painful, a special mouthwash containing lidocaine might help to control the symptoms.[93] Talk to your doctor or dentist about whether this would be an option for you.

Muscle/Joint Pain

It is a particularly ironic and perverse fact that the medication to control your RA can cause pain in your joints and muscles. "But aren't these meds supposed to deal with joint pain?" you may very well be asking. Well, yes and no. We take these kinds of medications to control our disease, not specifically to treat pain. When the meds work, they often bring about a decrease in pain because the inflammation of active RA has subsided. The meds working can also occasionally cause joint and muscle pain as a side effect.

In addition to RA, I also have fibromyalgia. When I was on Enbrel, it exacerbated my fibromyalgia, causing severe pain. Two years into taking the medication, my RA was well-managed, with no swelling and no further damage, but the muscle pain was limiting my life as much as active RA had done. My rheumatologist and I discussed it and decided to switch to Humira. I still get muscle (but not joint) pain after my shot of Humira, but it's much less than with Enbrel and only lasts a few days. In my book, temporary pain that can be managed is far better than the severe pain of active RA.

My reaction to Enbrel was unusually strong. Most people don't experience muscle pain at all, and for the ones that do, it usually abates within a few days of taking the medication. The even better news is that it's normally much less than the kind of pain you experience with active RA. Most importantly, it does not damage your joints.

If you do get this type of side effect, treat it like you would other types of pain. Take some painkillers and use heat or ice. For more pain management tools, see Part III: Pain Management Toolbox. Should you be among the small number of people who find their medication-related pain getting unreasonable and difficult to manage, talk to your doctor about exploring other types of treatment.

Shingles

Shingles is a painful rash or series of blisters that wraps around your torso on the left or right side. This condition is caused by the varicella-zoster virus, the same virus that causes chicken pox. When you've had chicken pox, the virus may lie dormant for years and be reactivated when you're an adult. You may be more vulnerable to developing shingles if you are over sixty, had chickenpox before the age of one or have a compromised immune system, such as from taking an immuno-suppressant for your RA. Having a case of shingles is not dangerous, but it can be quite painful.[94] It can also take quite a while to subside.

A review of studies presented at the annual EULAR meeting in 2012 show that people who are on anti-TNF drugs such as Enbrel, Humira or Remicade have a 75% higher risk of getting shingles than those treated with conventional DMARDs.[95] That can sound as if you are doomed to get shingles, but when translated, the facts are less scary. The rate of actual cases of shingles was found to be almost 5% in Germans treated with anti-TNF drugs and 20% in Americans treated with these medications.[96] Those numbers are a lot less likely to cause anxiety.

As with so many other side effects, awareness and preparation are key. If your doctor suggests that you take an anti-TNF medication, discuss the possibility of shingles with them. One way to manage the risk is to get the shingles vaccine before you start the medication — it can reduce the possibility of getting shingles by up to 50%.[97] If you're already taking an immunosuppressant drug, you should not get the shingles vaccine.

Being aware of the possible symptoms of shingles can help you get treatment as soon as possible, should you develop this condition. Antiviral drugs, such as Zovirax (acyclovir) and Valtrex (valacyclovir), can help you heal faster and reduce the risk of complications.[98] As well, if the pain from shingles is hard to deal with, a number of different medications may help control the symptoms. These include anticonvulsants such as Neurontin (gabapentin), numbing agents in cream, gel or spray form or narcotic painkillers. Taking a cool bath or using cold compresses on the rash may also soothe the pain and itching.[99]

This chapter covered a small and pretty random collection of potential side effects that didn't easily fit into another chapter. Some are fairly common side effects. Others are usually rare, but the kinds of side effects that a lot of people worry about (see above section on hair loss). The description of each was fairly short, intended to give you enough information to get started on more research if you need it. Keep the lines of communication open with your doctor, do enough research to be aware, but not so much that you freak out. Then remind yourself why you're taking the medication: to protect your body, to live your life. And then go do just that.

27
Rare and Serious Side Effects

aka "the scary chapter"

And now we come to the serious side effects, which thankfully are also in the rare category. Some of the side effects discussed in this chapter require pharmaceutical companies to label certain medications with what's called a black box warning. This means that studies have indicated the medication carries a risk of serious or even life-threatening side effects. These are the scary ones, the ones we all hope we'll never experience. And most of us won't. As you read this chapter, it's important to remember that — you will likely never get these types of side effects. However, being aware of their existence may help you prevent them or, should you be one of the few people who do develop a rare side effect, get on top of the situation straight away.

Although these side effects are rare, the reality is that some of us will experience them. We each have to come to terms with the risk in our own way. Do the research and talk to your rheumatologist about the actual statistics of how much of a risk you're taking and ways to minimize that risk. Once the reading and talking are done, you have to think. Think about what your life means to you. About what will happen if you do not take the medication, because that also carries risks. Eventually, you will get to a place where you're comfortable with your decision.

This chapter is by no means an exhaustive guide to the serious side effects of various RA medications. It will give it a short overview of a selected few. Some of these are what you might call the Big Bad, the ones that seem to leap off the list of side effects and hit that instinctive, unreasonable fear that interferes with sound decision-making. The good news is that if you develop certain of these rare and scary side effects, they will likely appear gradually. In some cases, stopping the medication may stop the progression of a particular side effect. Not all of them, though, and you have to face that risk with open eyes.

Ready?

Autoimmune Diseases

Oh joy, oh bliss. As if it wasn't enough to have RA, one of the rare side effects of certain of the biologics can be developing other autoimmune diseases such as lupus or multiple sclerosis (MS). When you research the meds suggested by your doctor, note whether other autoimmune diseases are listed as a possible side effects. If this is the case, make sure you know some of the basic symptoms of these conditions so you can recognize them if they happen.

As mentioned earlier in the book, one of the problems with informed consent is the development of a slight hypochondria problem. Knowing the symptoms of certain serious conditions can give you what's called "medical student syndrome." It's quite common for medical students to develop symptoms of whatever disease they are currently studying and this may happen to you, as well. For instance, one of the characteristic symptoms of lupus is what's called a butterfly rash on the face, covering both cheeks and the bridge of the nose. If you look a little rosy in this area, it's easy to jump to the conclusion that you have lupus, quickly followed by an episode of freaking out. Of course, the fact that you had a lovely lunch in the noonday sun by the water earlier in the day couldn't possibly be the explanation, could it?

Remember the mantra: these types of side effects are rare. The risk of you developing an autoimmune disease as a side effect to your medication is very low. There's a fine line between being aware of the possibility of a particular side effect and fretting over it on a daily basis. Remember that the medications are there to help you enjoy your life. If you notice a strange symptom, take a big step back, breathe deeply and approach it logically. If logic doesn't make your worry go away, call your doctor.

Birth Defects

Most people are aware that pregnancy and medication don't mix. A developing fetus can't have any chemical interference with its growth, so pregnant women do their very best to stay away from medication as much as possible.

Most RA meds are contraindicated for pregnancy. This means they're not good for the baby. If you're thinking of becoming pregnant, or you are sexually active and therefore might accidentally become pregnant, make sure you're aware of the implications of the medications you take. Talk to your rheumatologist about this issue to find out what the risks are and how to manage them. Some drugs should be avoided when trying to get pregnant, while others appear to be relatively safe. For instance, the effects of the biologics on the developing fetus are not yet known, but there seems to be growing evidence that it is safe to conceive while on, for instance, Enbrel.[100] However, most rheumatologists still recommend going off RA meds once you become pregnant. Even if you have discussed the issue with your doctor in a theoretical way, if you find out you're pregnant, call your rheumatologist right away.

A possible exception to the rule of no RA meds during pregnancy is prednisone. Although the majority of women go into remission when pregnant, for those who do not, prednisone is generally considered safe enough to help manage symptoms until the baby is born.

And now for the serious and scary part. Two RA meds are so dangerous to the developing fetus that it is essential you not get pregnant if you're taking them. Methotrexate and Arava cause severe birth defects. Throughout this book, I've tried to be as reassuring as possible, but not in this regard. The potential for severe birth defects is very real and should be taken seriously. You don't want to put yourself or your baby through that experience if it can be avoided.

If you take methotrexate or Arava, you *must* use effective birth control and preferably more than one kind. That means that if you have an IUD or use birth control pills, make sure your partner uses a condom, as well. Do not get "carried away," and do not leave home without condoms in your purse or pocket. This can be especially hard for women, because it's

149

not considered ladylike to plan for sex. I look at it this way: if you're old enough to have sex, you're old enough to be responsible about it. Both men and women should remember that it is possible to conceive any time during a woman's monthly cycle, including while she's having her period. Be careful — carry a condom.

If you take methotrexate or Arava and want to get pregnant, you will need to eliminate the drug from your body before you try to conceive. There are two approaches to doing this. One is to stop the medication and wait for a designated amount of time before trying to get pregnant. This allows your body to process the drug and eliminate it from your system. For women taking methotrexate, it is usually recommended to be off the medication for three to six months before trying to get pregnant. For Arava, some sources recommend up to two years between stopping the medication and trying to conceive. As well, some recommend pausing for two months between taking Arava and trying another type of RA medication.[101]

That's a very long time to wait. The second approach to making sure it's safe to try to get pregnant is to complete a washout regimen. This involves taking a medication called cholestyramine, a sort of antidote to Arava, for approximately eleven days. In an article in *Teratology* — a journal about the study of birth defects — Dr. Robert L. Brent recommends that all women of childbearing age who stop taking Arava undergo a drug elimination procedure (i.e., a washout regimen).[102] Taking cholestyramine is not an entirely pleasant experience — it can make you very nauseated — but it's better than waiting two years.

It is not known whether Arava can be passed on through semen to cause birth defects or fetal death if a man's partner becomes pregnant. However, to be on the safe side, Brent recommends that men who wish to father a child undergo the drug elimination procedure, as well.

Pretty nerve-racking, isn't it? Unfortunately, there is no way of sugarcoating the potential risk for severe birth defects. Make sure you discuss this aspect of treatment with your rheumatologist, so you can take precautions. If you're a woman taking methotrexate or Arava and you experience symptoms of possible pregnancy such as missed period, morning sickness or breast tenderness, contact your doctor immediately for advice.

Cancer

The C-word. Just seeing the word is enough to send off the *whoop, whoop, whoop* of an internal alarm, making you want to curl up in a corner, sucking your thumb.

The risk of developing cancer, and which type of cancer depends on the drug. When I first started Enbrel in 2005, it was thought to cause an increased risk of cancer. Subsequent studies have shown that taking one of the anti-TNF medications (Enbrel, Humira, Remicade) does not expose you to increased risk.[103] Other studies have shown that there is a somewhat heightened risk when you take higher doses of anti-TNF drugs. However, since RA itself is associated with an increased risk of cancer, it is uncertain whether this result is due to the medication or having RA.[104]

It's important that you and your rheumatologist discuss not just your own medical history, but also your family's. If you do have a family history of cancer, it may change your doctor's recommendations in terms of which drugs you should take.

When you discuss the option of a new medication with your doctor, it's a good idea to ask how much the drug might increase your risk. Often we hear the words "increased risk of cancer" and run the other way. In actual fact, the risk may be very low. Keeping your sense of perspective is essential. Remember that the risk may be less than that of being in a car accident and that most of us get in a car every day without thinking about it. It may also be that the possible benefits of the drug outweigh the risks. In 2005, that was the case for me. My RA was eating my life, and I had no quality of life. Therefore, the risk was worth it for me.

There are things you can do to manage the risk of cancer. Take precautions in general — eat a healthy, balanced diet, be as fit as you can be, use sunblock and so on. It's also a very good idea to get annual checkups such as Pap smears, mammograms, colonoscopies, prostate checks and mole checks. Talk to your family doctor about having a plan that would ensure early detection of any problems. If you develop cancer — whether caused by medication or not — early detection can be a very important factor in successful treatment.

Fungal Infections

The biologics leave you more vulnerable to developing infections, many of which are manageable and relatively benign. Most people have experienced sinus or bladder infections and although you may be more susceptible to getting these kinds of infections, they are easily treated. However, the biologic medications that are in the TNF alpha drug category — Enbrel, Humira, Remicade, Cimzia and Simponi — can also make you vulnerable to developing certain opportunistic fungal infections. One of these infections is histoplasmosis. This is an infection affecting the lungs, caused by a fungus called *Histoplasma capsulatum*. It behaves much like pneumonia, but may eventually spread to the bloodstream. At present, an enhanced warning appears on these medications regarding histoplasmosis. Recently, the FDA also added warnings pertaining to *Listeria* and *Legionella* bacteria.[105]

This doesn't mean that you should freak out because you're destined to get a really horrible infection. You're not — like the other side effects discussed in this chapter, the risk of developing frightening infections is very low. These warnings exist to make doctors more aware of the risk, so they can give you better care. Before the risk of histoplasmosis was known, a number of people died from the infection, primarily due to delayed diagnosis.[106] When doctors are more aware of the potential risk, these types of infections are much more likely to be caught quickly and treated effectively.

You should be aware that histoplasmosis in particular is more common in certain geographical areas. In the US, people who live in states near the Ohio River Valley and the lower Mississippi River should be particularly careful regarding this type of fungal infection.[107] North of the border, it is primarily found in central Canada. If you live in any of these areas, make sure you discuss the issue thoroughly with your rheumatologist and family doctor. When you and your care team are aware of this possibility, you will be better equipped to prevent such an infection or discover it early. This will help you get potentially life-saving treatment as soon as possible.

Liver Damage

Your liver is an important organ, responsible for a number of functions in the body including detoxification and digestive processes. It usually carries on fairly quietly, so most people don't pay any attention to it. This will change if you are on Arava or methotrexate.

Methotrexate is usually the first medication to be prescribed for RA, while Arava is used more rarely. These medications both have the potential to cause problems with the liver. More specifically, they can cause cirrhosis of the liver — a condition in which scarring replaces healthy tissues, causing the organ to malfunction — and liver failure.[108] In the summer of 2010, after more evidence of severe liver damage was found, the FDA required a strong warning to be issued on Arava packaging.[109] If you take one of these drugs, your doctor will order regular blood tests to monitor your liver function, usually every six weeks.

Because of the possibility of damage to your liver, your rheumatologist will tell you to drink alcohol very sparingly while you're on these meds. Some people find the idea of this very difficult and again, you have to weigh the pros and cons of treatment. For many, protecting joints, health and mobility outweighs giving up alcohol.

If you already have liver damage or are an alcoholic, it's generally not recommended that you take these drugs for your RA. That's stating it very bluntly, but it's necessary. Even if you have trouble facing the fact that you may have an addiction to alcohol, don't hide it from your doctor. There are other options for treating your RA and it is not worth the risk. Even if you enjoy a drink socially, make sure you talk to your rheumatologist about the risk associated with alcohol and the meds you take. Doing so means you have all the information you need to decide what to do when you're out with friends, at a Christmas party or toasting the bride and groom.

By now, even I am getting nervous, but keep in mind that all medications carry possible serious risks. As long as you take precautions, such as regular blood work and staying away from alcohol, methotrexate and Arava are reasonable options for treatment of RA. As is always the case, discuss the issue thoroughly with your rheumatologist before starting the medication to make sure you fully understand the pros and cons.

Tuberculosis

Years ago when I heard the word tuberculosis (TB), I thought of pale, terribly romantic people such as the poet Keats or any number of operatic heroines, slowly and prettily succumbing to consumption while coughing delicately into a handkerchief. Then my rheumatologist mentioned testing me for TB before I started Enbrel, and it didn't seem so romantic anymore.

Of course, actually having TB is nowhere near as pretty as the operas and books would have it. It is an infection of the lungs, causing fatigue, fever and coughing. In the past, people with TB would often waste away (hence the name consumption). Now it can be treated effectively with antibiotics. You may have heard of drug-resistant TB, where the disease doesn't respond to the medication. This is more common if the treatment isn't taken correctly — for instance, if the person does not take the TB meds regularly or doesn't finish the full course of treatment.[110]

Certain of the biologics, such as Enbrel and Humira, have been associated with developing tuberculosis, especially during the first year of treatment. Such cases are generally thought to be from a reactivation of latent TB, which means that the disease was already present in your body. Therefore, getting a TB test before you start these medications is essential. If you test negative, there's no reason to believe that you will develop tuberculosis.

This has been a long and scary chapter. The kind that makes you wish for the days when you just handed over decisions about your health to the doctor, instead of bothering with all that informed consent nonsense.

Informed consent is very much *not* nonsense and is an essential part of living with a chronic illness. It's scary at times, but there is a lot of truth in the adage that information is power. The more you know, the more in control of your life you are.

There's a very good chance that you'll progress with your treatment and your life without having to worry about serious health problems resulting from medication. But there's an unexpected side effect (if you will) to thinking about all of this. Being one of the few who have decided that the benefits of a particular path outweigh the possible risks involved does something a little special. Living with the awareness that you have deliberately chosen a road where the knife's edge is a little sharper than most people's has a way of bringing extra luster to your life. Never again will you take it for granted.

28

Side Effects Wrap-Up

"I'm overwhelmed."

Sixteen chapters describing different kinds of potential side effects is a lot. I hope you took my advice from the introduction in Chapter 11 and used this part of the book as a reference tool. Dipping in and out of these chapters as you need them is much less nerve-racking than reading all of them in one go.

This is probably a good time to remind you that any side effects you may have will likely be completely manageable. There are people on both extremes of the continuum, some who don't experience any side effects at all — lucky ducks — and some who get hit hard. For most, side effects become just part of the landscape.

When you look at your side effects, you have to ask yourself certain questions. Are they manageable? Is your life first, the disease and side effects second? Are you in a place where it's possible to laugh every day (even though it's sometimes a bit of gallows humor)? Quality of life is what determines the effectiveness of a medication and how reasonable side effects are. Should your side effects start to affect your quality of life as much as untreated RA, it's time to talk to your doctor to reassess your options. The goal of these medications is set you free, not to chain you in another way.

During the edit of this part of the book, I started thinking about what kind of side effects I've experienced during my four decades of living with RA. Looking back on the personal examples included in many of the chapters, there are quite a lot. I seem to be one of those people who react strongly to medication. Many of the side effects I've discussed are part of my current reality, including sinus problems, fatigue, fuzzy brain, dryness, gas, bloating, constipation, allergies, asthma, and the list goes on.

Realizing this was a little overwhelming and got me thinking about the cost of medication — the physical one, not the financial. There was a brief moment when it seemed to be a rather high cost. And then I shrugged and got on with my life.

Most of the time, side effects and managing them are second nature, just part of my life. Some of them are continuous, happening every day, some last for only a few days following my shot of Humira. Thankfully, they have lessened in intensity over time. Perhaps this is due to my body becoming used to the medication, perhaps it's because I've discovered ways of minimizing the side effects. Do I wish I didn't have to do this? Sure I do. But there is too much life to be lived out there. I've come to the conclusion that I can waste my time wishing that reality wasn't quite so real, or go out there and create a reality that makes it all worthwhile.

What it all boils down to is that when I look at my hand, I can see my knuckles. I have mostly manageable pain levels and my toes don't look like little sausages, swollen with inflammation. And it's about more than what it has done to manage my disease. Because of the medication, I can spend my life doing things like writing a book, helping others and laughing every day. And that means most of these side effects are more than worth it.

PART III:
PAIN MANAGEMENT
TOOLBOX

29
Pain Management Introduction

A big part of living well with RA is wrapping your head around the fact that there will likely be pain. No one likes to think about that. In fact, we'd all prefer that pain did not exist at all, wouldn't we?

Expecting your existence to be pain-free is the stuff of fairytales. Pain is part of life. You might even say that pain is a symptom of life. Many of the most interesting things that happen to us, the events that make us feel and make us grow, are accompanied by pain. Birth, heartbreak, disappointment and learning not to touch the stove when it's on — there's no getting through life without experiencing pain.

When you live with RA, pain is often a part of your reality. Even people who are diagnosed early and get their disease under control quickly will remember the pain from before the meds kicked in and may get sore if they push it too hard. Others who are not in remission or who have damage in their joints may have chronic pain.

There are different kinds of pain — the ache of overdoing it, the bone-deep hurting of a flare or the sharper pain that comes from damaged joints. Throughout your life with this disease, you may experience all of these and others, too. Increasingly, treatments work so well that more and more people experience very low levels of pain. Still, there may be times in your life with RA when there's a lot of pain, the kind that stops you from doing what you want. There may also be times when hurting is part of your daily life, but at a low enough level that you can get on with living. And that is exactly the goal of pain management: to give you the ability to engage with your life as fully as possible.

Getting to that place where your life is first and the pain is second needs more than medication. It can take a toolbox of coping mechanisms, ranging from lifestyle changes to adding a pain specialist to your care team. This section will introduce you to a number of different items to put in your toolbox. Used together, they can help you to focus on things other than the pain. Some are the more standard tools for managing pain, involving different types of professionals in the healthcare field, while others are tricks I've learned in the past forty plus years of living with RA.

One of the most important tools is your attitude, and you'll see that idea reflected in a number of the following chapters. The experience of pain can be paralyzing and can fill you with fear. Putting pain in perspective is the beginning to finding your way out of that fear. Coming to understand that pain isn't the worst thing that can happen — not living your life is — will help you more than you can imagine. Remember that, even if you have a lot of pain. Find some part of the day that belongs to you alone, that represents your life. It will help you fight back.

Another important tool is a sense of control. Living with a chronic illness that is characterized by a certain level of unpredictability can make you feel as if someone else is running your life. Not feeling in control can lead to feeling helpless, and when you feel helpless, you can become depressed. Finding a way to exert some level of control over your symptoms can help. By using medication and the tools in your pain management toolbox, you can get to a place where you're better able to cope. Once you realize that there are things you can do to prevent certain kinds of flares and to lower your pain levels, your strength comes back and the sense of control shifts from the disease to you. And therein lies your power.

30
Medicating Pain

"I should be able to deal with this."

"My doctor gave me a prescription for painkillers, but I only take them when I absolutely can't stand it anymore."
"My family worries that I take too many pills."
"I don't want to become addicted." (See Chapter 9.)

Do you recognize any of those statements? Convincing yourself to take the medications that suppress RA is one thing — there is very clear evidence that it is a sensible thing to do (see Chapter 3). It can be quite another to wrap your head around the idea of taking painkillers.

We grow up learning to be a big boy or girl when we fall and hurt ourselves, encouraged to buck up and not cry. This is the beginning of learning that our culture values toughness in the face of pain. Showing that you hurt or taking medication to cope is sometimes seen as a sign of weakness. On the other hand, bearing pain with no outward sign is admired. It's seen as being strong, and we all like to be strong, right?

Here's the thing about that — there is no objective way to measure pain. People who haven't experienced pain from surgery or medical conditions have no way of knowing what it is like to live inside the experience. Yet others often feel free to share their judgment of what you should be able to handle. And it's contagious. If you get enough of those messages, you start asking yourself if you should be able to handle the pain without help. And at the end of the road, there you are in the middle of an RA flare, trying to persuade yourself not to take painkillers.

Is that reasonable? There are some questions you can ask yourself to test whether your response is based in your own reality or in the myth that strength means you must bear pain without flinching.

Is your quality of life affected by your pain? Does the pain prevent you from doing things you have to do or would like to do? Does the pain affect your mood, making you sad or angry or frustrated? Does the pain affect your relationships, making you impatient with your kids or contributing to fights with your partner? Are you exhausted all the time because the pain is part of everything you do? And here's another question: if someone you love were in pain, the kind that colored every hour of their day, would you expect them to carry on as normal or would you hand them the painkillers and a glass of water?

Being in pain is an unreasonable state of being. Taking painkillers is a reasonable response to an unreasonable situation.

Winning the Race

The first step to managing your pain is to get your RA under control (see Chapters 3 and 4). Treating the disease and getting the inflammation under control will do wonders for your daily pain levels. In fact, it can take you to a point where you have hardly any pain at all. The treatment options available today mean that it is more possible than ever before to go into remission or have low disease activity. This means little or no inflammation, which vastly decreases pain levels and prevents damage to joints, thereby also preventing pain.

Some people, however, continue to have pain on a chronic basis. Sometimes, it's because they have trouble finding a medication that suppresses their RA. At other times, it is pain due to the damage that happened in the joints before the disease was controlled. Pain from damaged joints is a different quality of pain than that of active RA. It's sharper, cleaner somehow, but it's still pain that can impact your ability to get on with your life.

One of the first steps to learning how to manage your pain is a shift in how you think about it. When people experience acute, temporary pain such as a sprained ankle or a headache, they often wait to take medication until it's pretty bad. As long as you're dealing with a garden-variety headache or a fairly mild injury, there's nothing wrong with that approach.

When you have chronic pain on the other hand, you need to deal with it in a completely different way. You are in a race with your pain. Waiting until you can't take it anymore means the medication will only take the top off your pain. That can lead to you always having high levels of unreasonable pain. A better solution is taking the pain meds at regular intervals so that you will always have medication in your system. Therefore, the meds will deal with all or most of your pain, not just the tip of the iceberg.

The different types of medications that manage pain are outlined in Chapter 5. How you use these meds can vary and usually takes some tinkering, listening to your body's messages and trying different ways of taking the painkillers.

Most prescriptions for painkillers will indicate an appropriate interval on the label, for instance, "take every six hours or as needed." That means that it is safe for you to take the medication every six hours, but not more than that. If taking your medication as it is prescribed helps you get through the day, be able to participate in your life and enjoy what you do, go ahead and do so. If you are able to do what you need to do and enjoy your life with less medication, the "as needed" is an indication that you can reduce how frequently you take the meds. The key to determining what you need is going back to the mantra: can you live your life and enjoy it? If the answer is yes, you're good. If the answer is no, even when taking the medication at the interval suggested on the prescription, talk to your doctor about increasing the dose or perhaps adding stronger pain meds (see Chapter 5).

When you have chronic pain, the race starts even before you wake up — morning pain and stiffness that can take a long time to subside are common symptoms of RA. As a child, I spent a lot of time in a rehab hospital, and the nurses taught me a very useful trick to make mornings tolerable that I still use to this day. Set your alarm clock to a couple of hours before you have to get up, take your pain meds, eat a piece of apple or a couple of crackers to make sure the meds don't hurt your stomach and go back to sleep. By the time you have to get up, the painkillers are working and this makes facing the day much less intimidating. Following through with pain medication throughout the day will keep you ahead of the pain and help you focus on what's really important.

The bottom line is that when you live with chronic pain, you have to break with conventions, be they spoken or unspoken. You learn to assess stereotypes and social myths not in terms of "what everyone knows," but in terms of whether they make sense in your life. Sucking up the kind of pain that interferes with your quality of life and makes it hard to be part of your community, your work and your family is not going to result in recognition or reward. It just gets you weeks or months of watching everyone else move on with their life. That might sound a bit blunt, but bucking convention takes plain speaking. The myth that painkillers are for wimps was created by people who didn't have chronic pain.

So take the meds. And go live your life.

31
Pain Management Specialists

"Can't someone help me get rid of this pain?"

When you talk to your rheumatologist about pain control, they may tell you that they treat inflammation, not pain. It's hard to understand — after all, if someone specializes in a disease that historically has come with chronic pain, you'd think pain management would be part of the package. However, it is the point of view of many rheumatologists that if they treat the pain, it could mask the symptoms of RA and therefore increase the risk of permanent damage to your joints.

Keep in mind that with early diagnosis and treatment, many people can go into remission or experience low disease activity. This can mean that they'll never need a pain specialist. Other people may get their pain management needs met through the existing members of their medical team, including their rheumatologist (some will prescribe pain medication) and family doctor. However, people who have trouble getting their RA suppressed, have significant damage or have trouble getting adequate pain control may benefit from seeing someone who specializes in treating chronic pain. There is an increasing understanding that pain is a complex process of neurological responses, a condition in and of itself instead of just a symptom. Therefore, pain requires as much study and knowledge as any other illness.[111]

Enter the pain management specialist.

Finding a good pain specialist can be a bit of a challenge. At this time, there is no officially recognized pain specialty in the US or Canada, so theoretically, any doctor can claim to be a pain specialist.[112] Getting a referral from your rheumatologist or family doctor means that the pain specialist will have been "prescreened" by them as a legitimate and experienced pain specialist. As well, pain management programs may be run through hospitals or rehab clinics. This is also a stamp of approval.

When you have the first appointment, come prepared with a list of questions to make sure that you and the treatment approach used will mesh and therefore be more effective. Examples of topics to discuss can include the doctor's background and how they came to specialize in pain management. You can also ask about the kinds of treatments they offer — are they primarily focused on medication or do they favor a multidisciplinary approach? If medication is part of their practice, talk about their position on treatment agreements (see Chapter 9).

Talking about the dynamic between you and the pain specialist will give you an idea of whether they view the process as a partnership or a more traditional doctor-patient relationship in which you are expected to comply with their recommendations. Some people like to bring a friend or family member to appointments for moral support and to help remember everything that happened. If having a wingman would make you more comfortable, it's important that the doctor embraces this dynamic. And lastly, you'll want to talk about the kind of outcome they envision for the treatment — do they promise you the moon or are they more realistic in their expectations? As in the case of infomercials, if what they say sounds too good to be true, you may want to be a bit skeptical.

Asking questions will not only gives you a sense of where the doctor's coming from, but also reveals their level of comfort in working with an engaged pain patient. Ideally, you'll want to find someone who will work with you as a team and empower you to deal with your pain, not someone who wants you to do what they tell you without question.

The approach of pain specialists can vary greatly. Some doctors focus on managing the prescription and administration of pain medication, including opioids and other painkillers. These kinds of drugs can be an essential tool in helping to manage your pain. However, when you're dealing with chronic pain, relying solely on medication excludes other techniques that can be valuable contributors to living well with your pain. Pain management that incorporates a multidisciplinary treatment approach can be much more effective than medication alone.

In addition to medication management, a multidisciplinary approach to treatment of pain can include physical and occupational therapy, massage, biofeedback, meditation, counseling, peer support groups, as well as other services. Some pain management programs will include all the services under one roof, but sometimes you'll have to add certain other treatments yourself. At the end of the day, when used together, these different types of treatments can teach you how to live well with your pain.

To be successful, pain treatment depends not just on what your specialist and their team do, but also on you. An essential aspect of responding well to such treatment is to manage your expectations. Do enough research about your condition by reading books and websites so you know the boundaries you may be facing. For instance, if you experience a significant amount of pain from damaged joints, expecting your doctor or a pain program to make your life pain-free may set you up for failure. In such a situation, a more realistic goal may be manageable pain and a significantly increased quality of life.

It's important to realize that this is a process that will take time. You'll likely have to try different things before you find the combination that works. By the time you see a pain specialist, you may have been in a lot of pain for a long time, and this can make you feel quite desperate and hopeless. Have faith that together, you and the pain management team will get you to a place where you have healthy coping skills and manageable pain.

It is possible.

32
Heat and Ice

"Ahhhh, that's better..."

"Why is your butt cold?"

These charming words came from my partner during a romantic moment at the beginning of our relationship. His hand had wandered down my back to lovingly caress my derrière, only to stop, move back to warmer climes and look at me with question marks in his eyes.

I have an ice pack at my back at all times. Sitting in a wheelchair for a full day is hard on your body, particularly your lower back. Several years ago, I discovered that placing an ice pack between it and the back of my wheelchair helped control pain and offered a bit of added support. The downside is that my rear end often has the temperature of an icicle.

Heat and ice treatments have been used for ages to treat pain — both are wonderful tools that can be very effective in reducing your pain levels. Will heat or ice work best for you? The only way to tell is to give them a try. To make everything even more confusing, what works best can depend on the part of your body that's hurting or the reason you're in pain. For instance, an injury such as a sprained ankle or pulled muscle often responds better to ice. In fact, it is generally recommended that you treat such an injury with ice for the first two days and then alternate between heat and ice.

There are no specific recommendations to treat RA-related pain, whether it's from active inflammation or damaged joints. Some people respond very well to heat, while others say it makes their joints feel more inflamed. Likewise, some people enjoy ice packs and, for others, they make the pain worse. Sometimes ice works great one day and heat better the next. Play around with both to get a sense of what's most effective for you under which circumstances.

Heat

Wrapping heat around aching joints lets it seep into your bones and muscles, easing stiffness and leaving nothing but relaxation behind. It can be positively blissful.

There are numerous ways of warming up your joints. One of the easiest is to use a heating pad or heat therapy bags that are heated in the microwave. Both heating pads and bags are available at most drugstores. You can also make the bags yourself by sewing tubes of material into varying lengths and filling them with rice, corn or grain. Store-bought bags have recommendations on the packaging for how long they should be in the microwave before they're ready. If you use homemade bags, err on the side of caution when you first heat them to avoid cooking the contents. One other note of caution: when you use these kinds of tools, be careful not to get things too hot and burn your skin. Placing the bag or heating pad directly on the skin may not be a good idea. Put it on top of a clothed part of your body or place a towel between you and the heating pad or bag.

You can also treat pain in your hands and feet by sinking them into a warm paraffin bath. A paraffin bath is a container in which you melt cakes of paraffin wax and then soak the body part in question for twenty minutes or so. They're often used at spas for manicures, as they make your skin as soft as a baby's bottom. Paraffin baths can be a wonderful tool to ease the pain of RA. As you soak your hands for instance, you'll find that the paraffin starts building up a large, soft glove. It can take a bit of getting used to but is sort of fun, as well. When your time's up, you scrape off the wax, and it can usually be reused. If this sounds like something you'd like to try, search for "paraffin bath" online in places like Amazon or check with your local drugstore.

This one is going to sound weird, but it's worked for me since I was a little girl. If you're having a really rough time with say, a wrist, try wrapping it in soft plastic such as cling wrap. Add a wrist warmer or cotton glove, a sock if it's your ankle, a pair of warm pajama pants if it's a knee and so on. Then let your joints bake for a couple of hours or even overnight. When I was a child, I'd often wear plastic on affected joints as I slept. In the morning, I'd peel off the sweaty pieces, feeling better. There's something about the heat and the sweating that comes with being wrapped in plastic that can improve your pain levels. I have no idea why — I just know it works.

Baking yourself (so to speak) in various ways can be tremendously helpful. Just as sweating out the pain in the joint can make it feel better, so can surrounding your entire body with heat to the point of sweating. It can feel as if you're releasing the pain and tension with every drop of sweat. Some people find warm pools, hot tubs and saunas very useful in dealing with their pain. Others say that this kind of humid heat makes them feel more inflamed. Again, the only way to find what works for you is to try it.

Baking in the sun has always made me feel better — it's as if the warmth of the sun seeps into my bones. The benefits may be a combination of the heat, the vitamin D from the sun and letting myself sit quietly and relax. If this works for you, keep in mind that you need to protect your skin from the harmful rays of the sun. This is especially true if you take medications that may cause photosensitivity (see Chapter 21). Apply a broad spectrum sunblock, wear a hat and cover up. You can still heat yourself up in the sun without risking skin damage.

And speaking of warmth, keeping warm in general can be very helpful. Buy an electric blanket and curl up under it while watching TV. Invest in some warm, woolen socks for your feet to warm up your ankles and toes. If your hands get stiff, especially in the winter or during the height of air conditioning season, a pair of fingerless gloves or wrist warmers can make a huge difference. Do you know someone who knits? Ask them to make socks or wrist warmers for you out of yummy, soft yarn, or if you knit yourself, there are plenty of easy, free patterns on the Internet. Put on a sweater, swirl a fancy scarf around your neck and warm up. It'll make your body feel better.

Ice

Most people shudder at the thought of ice packs — the idea of putting something that's come straight from the freezer on your body just seems wrong. However, ice can be very effective in reducing the feeling of heat that comes with inflammation. The cold sensation only lasts a short while, followed by a quite paradoxical feeling of warmth, as well as relief from the pain.

Ice is a lot more straightforward than heat and comes pretty much only in one form: something bendable from the freezer. You can buy ice packs in different sizes for very reasonable prices in most pharmacies. Stock up so you have several ready to use in your freezer. If you're caught without ice packs, a bag of frozen peas or corn will do the trick nicely. It doesn't matter what kind of frozen produce you use, as long as it's a bag of something small and sort of round. This makes it easy to wrap around an elbow, knee or other bendable joint.

To use an ice pack (or bag of peas), first wrap it in a dish towel or regular towel. Placing an ice pack directly on bare skin can be very uncomfortable and may even cause frostbite. Once wrapped, apply the ice pack to the part of your body that hurts, either laying it flat or bending it around the joint. Make sure you're comfortable and sit or lie down quietly for twenty minutes or so. You can apply ice longer than that, but make sure that your skin is doing OK. If it hurts, feels uncomfortable or your skin gets too cold, take a break.

I've met a few people over the years who don't feel an effect from either ice or heat, but they are in the minority. Most people will get relief from one or the other or maybe even both. If you are not dealing with an injury, there are no hard and fast rules about what to do. As with almost everything else, remember the mantra: play around with it until you discover what works for you.

33

Acupuncture

"I don't like needles and you're going to stick seventeen of 'em in me??"

Mention acupuncture and some people look at you as if you just grew an extra head. The idea that sticking needles into one part of your body can help pain in another part can seem illogical. Still, a lot of people consider acupuncture an important part of their pain management program. So what's all the fuss about?

I was about twelve years old the first time I tried acupuncture. It was the mid-1970s, and my family and I still lived in Denmark. I was a patient at a rehab hospital along with many other kids who had juvenile rheumatoid arthritis. Every weekend, I'd go home in a wheelchair, and every Monday morning, my mother would take me for an acupuncture treatment and then back to the hospital. Once there, I'd walk into the children's ward, my mother pushing the wheelchair behind me. Despite the evidence right in front of them, the medical staff continued to scoff at the idea of acupuncture, but their opinion didn't matter to us. What mattered was that it worked. For decades, acupuncture has been an essential part of my personal toolbox, easing symptoms of inflammation and dealing effectively with pain.

Acupuncture is a treatment that originated in Traditional Chinese Medicine over 2,500 years ago.[113] In this treatment, very thin needles are inserted in various points on the body. These points follow what are called meridians, channels carrying qi (pronounced "chi"), the life force. Chinese medicine posits that illnesses and physical problems originate in too much of one or more of four factors: damp, dry, heat and cold. Where the acupuncture needles are inserted depends on which aspect needs to be addressed in which part of the body. Sometimes the needle is inserted near the problematic area and sometimes in a completely different part of the body. According to Chinese medicine, rheumatoid arthritis is deemed to be the result of too much damp heat, and when you've lived inside a flare, this makes a lot of sense. To me, active RA has always felt soggy and hot.

One of the great things about acupuncture is that you don't have to fully embrace the philosophy behind it in order for treatments to work. In fact, it is no longer just practiced by people specializing in Traditional Chinese Medicine. Increasingly, it is also used in Western-based practices by doctors, chiropractors and physical therapists and is covered by many insurance plans.

The treatments don't hurt — the needles are so thin you can barely feel them going in. Once they have been inserted, you are left lying comfortably for about twenty minutes to let them do their thing. Although you don't have to buy into the philosophy behind Chinese medicine, I've found it helpful to engage in visualization during treatment, imagining the meridians being cleared of debris so the energy can flow freely. Doing so can help you enter a sort of meditative state of deep relaxation, which may help the process along. It also allows you to feel as if you're participating actively in your own healing, which is another way of feeling a bit more in charge of your health.

The pain-relieving effects of acupuncture can be either cumulative or temporary, depending on what condition is being treated. When used to treat an injury, the need for acupuncture stops when the injury has healed. However, in a chronic illness such as RA, the pain relief you get from acupuncture tends to be temporary. Therefore, regular treatments have a better chance of helping to keep you on an even keel.

In my experience, acupuncture can be tremendously helpful. However, occasionally it doesn't work and can even exaggerate the pain you already have. Sometimes this is related to the skill of the practitioner, so being careful in your search for an acupuncturist will increase your chances of finding a good one (see below).

Even when you find a very good acupuncturist, there may still be days when your body just doesn't want to cooperate. The way you respond to a particular treatment can differ from day to day, whether it's acupuncture, physical therapy or taking painkillers. Communicating how you respond to treatment — both in general and regarding specific needles — can help your practitioner adjust treatment to accommodate your body's needs.

Acupuncture has very definitely changed since my childhood. It's been astonishing to watch the attitudes of medical professionals change from scoffing to acceptance, even learning acupuncture so they can provide their patients with better care. Given how much acupuncture can contribute to the management of RA symptoms and pain, this development is very welcome indeed.

Finding an Acupuncturist

As with any treatment, it's important to find someone who knows what they're doing. If Western-based medicine makes you more comfortable, choose a practitioner such as a medical doctor, chiropractor or physical therapist who has taken a course in acupuncture. If you're comfortable looking into alternative medicine, you have a number of other options, as well. Doctors of naturopathic medicine receive training in acupuncture as part of their four-year degree. You can also find a doctor of Traditional Chinese Medicine, who typically receives a more in-depth education in the field of acupuncture.

In the US, the American Board of Medical Acupuncture provides certification of medical doctors who include acupuncture in their practice. The organization maintains a list of certified members and their locations, which may include a doctor in your area (www.dabma.org/ physicians.asp). You can find a licensed doctor of naturopathic medicine through the American Association of Naturopathic Physicians (www.naturopathic.org). This website also contains more information about naturopathic medicine, which you may want to consider as a way to improve your general health. In Canada, you can find information about naturopathic medicine, as well as search for a naturopath, on the site of the Canadian Association of Naturopathic Doctors (www.cand.ca). If you want to explore the field of Chinese medicine to see what it has to offer in addition to acupuncture, Acupuncture.com maintains a list of doctors of Traditional Chinese Medicine.

The Acupuncture Foundation of Canada Institute offers membership to licensed acupuncturists in a number of different professions, not just in Canada, but in the US and other countries across the world (www.afcinstitute.com). Members include medical doctors, doctors of Traditional Chinese Medicine, physical therapists, chiropractors, dentists and so on. This foundation also has a search function through which you can find a practitioner in your area.

There are numerous ways of finding someone who can give you acupuncture, but the first thing you need to know when looking for a practitioner of alternative medicine is what kind of legislation or regulation governs the field. This can help protect you by making sure the person treating you has the proper licenses and certifications needed to practice. As with many other forms of treatment in the alternative medicine field, the approach to regulation of acupuncture varies by area. Individual US states differ in their approach to certification requirements — some have passed laws, others have not. You can find out more about individual state laws on Acupuncture.com.

In Canada, acupuncture laws and regulations differ by province. For instance, British Columbia passed the Traditional Chinese Medicine Practitioners and Acupuncturists Regulation in 2001. In 2006, Ontario passed the Traditional Chinese Medicine Act.

It's worth doing a bit of digging on Google to find out what regulations govern the practice of acupuncture in your area. Use that information to interview the practitioner you choose about their qualifications before you decide to become a pincushion.

34

Massage and Touch

"Yes, that's the spot..."

"I love you."

This tender moment was not between me and my beloved, but rather between me and my shiatsu massage therapist. She'd just finished working through my body, putting pressure on specific points, occasionally in that *hurts so good* way. As usual, the treatment had ended with her gliding her fingers gently over my forehead, through my hair and pulling on my earlobes. As usual, it had been blissful. In fact, it was so wonderful, I felt compelled to express my appreciation. Since I was relaxed to the point that my brain wasn't really working, the words came out sort of unfiltered. She laughed quietly, used to me professing my love for her at the end of a treatment.

Massage has been used for thousands of years all over the world to improve physical and emotional healing by hands-on manipulation of muscles and soft tissue. It works by drawing blood flow to the area of your body that's being massaged. This "improves circulation by bringing oxygen and other nutrients to body tissues."[114] Massage can "help heal damaged muscle, stimulate circulation, clear waste products via the lymphatic system, boost the activity of the immune system, reduce pain and tension, and induce a calming effect."[115] Receiving a massage also reduces stress hormones and releases endorphins. I'm sure you've heard about endorphins — they're brain chemicals that act like opioids, such as morphine and codeine. Call them natural happy drugs that work really well for pain control.

Massage can be very beneficial for people with RA. It can help reduce morning stiffness, pain and the anxiety that often comes with living with an unpredictable chronic illness. In general, this type of therapy is considered most effective when used as a series of treatments, followed by maintenance treatments that can keep you ahead of the pain.[116]

Massage isn't always the right thing to do and is not recommended at all for certain conditions. It's therefore important that your massage therapist knows about your entire medical history, not just the issues related to your RA. As well, massage is contraindicated in specific local problems, such as an acute RA flare. If, for instance, your knee is flaring, the massage therapist can still work on the rest of your body, but should avoid massaging near the affected joint.[117]

There are many different types of massage therapy, but it may be helpful to think of them as divided into two types: Western and Eastern. In the Western tradition, certified or registered massage therapists are trained in a variety of techniques. Their treatments may be covered by insurance plans.

In order to be certified, the therapist has to complete training that in most areas consists of a minimum 500 hours, pass national board exams and be licensed or registered.[118] To find a certified massage therapist in the US, contact the American Massage Therapy Association (www.amtamassage.org). In Canada, do an Internet search for "registered massage therapist" and the name of your province to find your provincial association of massage therapists. If you're not in the US or Canada, finding out what regulations govern massage therapy in your country should be fairly easy. Enter "registered massage therapist" and the name of your country or region in the search engine of your choice (Google, Bing, Yahoo). Your doctor or physical therapist may also be able to give you tips on finding a massage therapist.

Regardless of which type of massage you choose, be aware that it can be quite intense. Be sure to keep the lines of communication open throughout your treatment so your massage therapist can adjust the pressure to suit you. Sometimes the aftereffects of massage can make you quite sore, so you may also want to consider starting with a light treatment. If you start light and build up gradually over several sessions, you're less likely to hurt after your treatment.

Therapeutic Touch

Therapeutic Touch, or integrative touch, is a very gentle form of massage that just barely touches the skin. It was originally developed in the 1970s as part of nursing care. It's a "noninvasive, holistic approach to healing which stimulates the receiver's own recuperative powers. It is a modern form of laying-on-of-hands and is based on principles of an energy exchange between people."[119] Many consider it one of the flakier healing practices. In my experience, though, it can be a wonderful aid to reduce pain and help you relax, especially when you're going through a rough time.

Many areas have programs that teach Therapeutic Touch. As it is not yet regulated by government agencies, do your research before you decide on a practitioner. In the US, you can find practitioners on the website of the Therapeutic Touch International Association (www.therapeutic-touch.org). In Canada or other countries, do an Internet search for "therapeutic touch" and the name of your province, region or country.

Shiatsu

Shiatsu therapy represents the Eastern tradition of massage therapy and is often used as part of Traditional Chinese Medicine. It is based on the same principles as acupuncture (see Chapter 33). Instead of inserting needles, a shiatsu therapist will apply gentle pressure on specific points along the meridians to unblock the channels and allowing qi to flow freely.

To find a trained and registered shiatsu therapist in the US, contact the American Organization for Bodywork Therapies of Asia (www.aobta.org). In Canada, the Shiatsu School of Canada Inc. maintains a list of practitioners who have graduated from the school (www.shiatsucanada.com). You can also look in your Yellow Pages or do an Internet search. Outside of North America, start with an Internet search.

Reiki

Reiki is a Japanese technique that integrates the idea of enabling the life force to flow freely with a gentle laying-on-of-hands to foster relaxation and promote healing.[120] It's a very holistic treatment that includes your physical, emotional and spiritual well-being and can be very helpful when you live with RA. If you're very sore, this is also a terrific alternative to more touch intensive treatments, such as massage or shiatsu therapy.

You can find a Reiki practitioner on the website of the International Center for Reiki Training (www.reiki.org). Based in the US, it teaches practitioners all over the world and may list someone qualified in your region. In Canada, you can find practitioners through the Canadian Reiki Association (www.reiki.ca) or through an Internet search.

The Touch of a Loved One

The healing qualities of touch aren't limited to certified therapists. Finding relief and relaxation can be as close your family, friends or partner.

When people who love you see that you're in pain, they'll often ask "what can I do?" At the same time, they might be afraid to touch you because you're hurting. This can make you feel very alone at a time when you need others the most. Tell your loved ones about touch and light massage. Let them know that this is one of the ways they can help you feel better, physically and emotionally.

Touching among lovers, partners and spouses isn't just limited to what you get up to when you're naked. We hold hands, caress each other's faces, let our fingers dance along each other's arms, backs and knees. Sometimes we're barely conscious of reaching out to touch, but at other times we try to relieve tight muscles in a shoulder. Ask your beloved for help when

181

your muscles and joints ache. They can give you a light massage, easing tensed muscles. They can also slide their hands across your skin or through your hair, leaving relaxation in their wake. Sometimes, just putting a warm hand on the place that hurts can trigger a domino effect of feeling safe and relaxed. And best of all, the touch of someone who loves you doesn't just help relieve pain — it also builds connection and intimacy that can bring you closer together.

People who aren't lovers don't touch each other a lot in our culture. However, the kinds of touch you use to ease pain do not cross the line between nonsexual and sexual. That means that family and friends can also help when your muscles are tense and your joints ache. Make sure both of you are comfortable in giving and receiving this kind of touch. If you've never been very touchy-feely before, start slowly and stay away from areas that are usually reserved for the touch of a lover (chest to mid-thigh). If it feels awkward for either of you, ask them to help in other ways. It's just as important to cook a meal, drive you to the doctor or just listen when you need a shoulder to cry on.

There are a variety of options available within the field of massage therapy. Which should you choose? In my experience, no one approach is better than another. You may respond better to Reiki than traditional Western massage techniques, or maybe it's the other way around. Try a few, see what you like. The most important factor in making the experience a good one is to communicate well with the therapist. Make sure they know what kinds of medical conditions you have and where you hurt before the session starts. During the session, let them know if something doesn't feel good so they can adapt to your needs. And if you find yourself professing your love for them, you know you've found a good one!

35

Meditation

"Ommmm..."

My first exposure to meditation was in the late 1970s when I took a course in Transcendental Meditation. It's a somewhat esoteric spiritual practice established in the 1950s by Maharishi Mahesh Yogi.[121] They claimed you could learn to fly. I never made it that far.

Although meditation never got me to levitate, it has helped me to be more grounded. I've learned that sitting quietly and stilling my mind is a terrific way to feel more at peace with the world and my place in it. Meditation also relaxes tense muscles and helps me build energy. Over the years, the techniques I use have changed and adapted to different situations in my life. What hasn't changed is that I still use meditation to quiet my mind, ease stress and control pain.

Many pain management clinics and programs incorporate meditation training as an important tool in coping with pain and the stress of living with a chronic illness. When you meditate on a regular basis, you teach your brain to focus on the present, which means you spend less time dreading future pain. Focusing on the present makes it easier to reduce the fear and the risk of depression that can happen when you anticipate potentially negative events such as RA flares. In other words, you may have pain, but the emotional experience of the pain has less of an impact.[122]

There are many forms of meditation, but what they all have in common is spending some time focusing and clearing your mind. Some people meditate by gazing at a candle flame, some by listening to ambient sound like the slow ringing of a bell or a CD with calming sounds from nature. Some forms of meditation use a mantra that is chanted out loud or repeated silently in your mind. Prayer can be a form of meditation, as can walking a labyrinth. For that matter, sitting on a park bench in the sunshine with your eyes closed and your heart open can be meditative, as well.

The kind of meditation taught in pain management and stress management courses is often associated with mindfulness training. This is a concept developed by Western psychology from Buddhist practice, but separated from its spiritual background. As applied to serious or chronic illnesses, mindfulness was pioneered by Jon Kabat-Zinn, founding director of the Stress Reduction Clinic at the University of Massachusetts Medical School.

Mindfulness can be defined as "paying attention in a particular way; on purpose, in the present moment and nonjudgmentally."[123] It can be a remarkable way to live your life. In my experience, it can do wonders for your emotional health and your ability to connect to joy and beauty. It takes practice, but when you do it on a regular basis, life gets much, much better, even during the rough times. An in-depth discussion of mindfulness is beyond the scope of this book. If you want to know more, Kabat-Zinn's book *Full Catastrophe Living: Using the Wisdom of Your Body and Mind to Face Stress, Pain, and Illness* and his audio program *Mindfulness for Beginners* are both excellent. They also include several lessons in meditation.

I highly recommend that you look into adding meditation to your pain management toolbox. Pick up Kabat-Zinn's books, take more in-depth lessons on meditation in a pain or stress management program or find another place that teaches meditation.

Most people react to such recommendations by putting it on their mental list and then forgetting about it. In case that's you, I'll share two easy approaches to meditation that you can start yourself. Give them a try. I bet you'll like them.

Both types of meditation involve sitting quietly for twenty minutes or so in a comfortable chair. Comfortable, but preferably not reclined — the goal is for you to focus, not to fall asleep. If you can't get comfortable in a chair, pick a position that feels good, even if it's lying down on your bed.

Try to meditate in the beginning or middle of your day. In the evening, you may be too tired and therefore more likely to fall asleep. If the evening is the only time you have, do whatever works for you. Once you're in a comfortable position, close your eyes and breathe. What happens next depends on which approach you'd like to try.

The first type is mindfulness-based meditation. In this kind of meditation you focus on your breathing and on merely observing your thoughts instead of engaging with them. This technique recognizes that you can't stop the thoughts from coming. If you have a random thought going by about needing to buy oranges, paying a bill or wondering what your teenager is up to, just watch them go by. Don't start thinking about other things to put on your grocery list or your bank balance, and you can probably benefit from a twenty-minute break from worrying about your teenager.

Remember the quote about paying attention to the moment nonjudgmentally? There is no wrong way of doing this. People who have meditated for decades still have thoughts flitting through their minds. They still instinctively follow them and still have to practice coming back to a place where they're not engaging with all the stuff that happens in their brains. One of the best ways of summing up this type of meditation is this:[124]

- Sit Down
- Don't move
- Shut up

Much easier said than done, but if you can do that for twenty minutes a day, you'll be way ahead. Don't think you have twenty minutes in your busy schedule? Start with five. You'll probably enjoy it so much that you'll find more time.

The other type of meditation that's worked very well for me was a technique I learned in a pain management program in the mid-1980s and still use. It also starts with sitting comfortably with your eyes closed. It differs from mindfulness-based meditation by including a visualization exercise to help modify your pain levels.

You start by getting physically comfortable and taking a few minutes to just sit and clear your mind, much like in mindfulness-based meditation. After a few minutes, you begin to create a place in your mind where you feel safe. It can be a memory from childhood, such as your grandmother's garden. It can also be a special spot you make up in your imagination like a waterfall in a tropical forest. What the place is doesn't matter. What matters is that you feel safe, secure and relaxed when you visit it in your mind.

After you have settled on your special place, spend some time filling in the details, such as what you see, feel, hear and smell. Once you're well established within the image and feel relaxed, warm and safe, imagine a depiction of your body in front of you. Perhaps it's on a magical blackboard or projected from the laptop that somehow appeared next to you. On the image of your body, create a representation of your pain in the area that hurts. Some people use the color red to denote inflammation, while others imagine a tightly wound spring. You get the idea. Again, there is no right or wrong, as long as it makes sense to you.

And now for the really interesting part. Change the pain on the projected image of your body. If you chose the color red, try slowly changing it to something non-hot like blue to cool the inflammation or erase it all together. If you chose a tightly wound spring, try to relax it into an overcooked piece of limp spaghetti. If what you chose doesn't help you change the pain despite it making sense in your mind, don't worry. Continue sitting quietly in a relaxed frame of mind, looking at the mental image of your body. Chances are that something will come to you. Once it does, you'll notice the pain easing. Through the visualization, you can learn to exert more control over something that previously seemed uncontrollable.

Of the two approaches to meditation I described, only one seems to deal specifically with pain. So why bother trying any other approach?

Living with RA can be a stressful experience. Balancing everything that goes into having a chronic illness, such as medical appointments, education, energy management and dealing with random flares means you're always alert and engaged. Trying to stay one step ahead is stressful. Stress, regardless of its source, often exacerbates pain and fatigue and makes it more difficult to cope.

Meditation, whether it involves visualization, chanting or mindfulness, can be tremendously helpful in reducing stress and the experience of pain, thereby helping you cope better. It can teach you how to be more in touch with your body, to connect to the physical part of you that many of us block out because it's a source of pain. This connection does not make you more aware of the pain, but rather puts it in perspective and helps you feel more in control.

Meditation may not make you fly, but it can make you feel more grounded and joyful. Give yourself the gift of twenty minutes of quiet every day. You won't regret it.

36
Managing Your Energy

"I'm so tired of being tired."

You've just gotten up from a full night's sleep and feel exhausted. You drag yourself to work and by lunchtime, you're achy and need a nap. Somehow, you manage to push through the afternoon, but by the time you get home, your joints are screaming and all you can do is keel over into bed.

Having RA often means having less energy. The disease itself causes a healthy dollop of fatigue, especially when it is not under control, and pain is very draining, too. RA-related fatigue isn't just being tired, it's being exhausted and it can start the minute you get up in the morning. Pain and fatigue are the evil twins of RA — being in pain takes a lot of energy — and when you have less energy, you feel the pain more. Learning how to manage your energy and working within your limits can be effective tools to manage pain and prevent flares.

For many of us, managing the fatigue that comes with RA is one of the most challenging aspects of living with the disease. It's one thing to read about fatigue, it's quite another to live with the consequences. Your house is a mess, you haven't cooked a proper meal in weeks and, if you're in pain, it makes you want to cry. Despite the mess, it's essential to learn to pay attention not to the tasks of the day, but instead to your body's opinion of them.

We are so used to living under pressure and to being in constant motion that the idea of doing only what is good for our bodies is something we plan to do when we retire. Backing off and doing less, either because you can't physically do what's required or because you choose to slow down, can feel like giving up or being lazy. Sometimes those around you also notice and join in what can only be described as a judgment party. Not only is the voice in your head berating you for slowing down, but sometimes the people in your life start questioning you, too.

How do you explain to both yourself and those around you the changes that living with a chronic illness have made?

A brilliant woman named Christine Miserandino invented the Spoon Theory to do just that. Having a meal in a diner with a friend, the subject of what it's like to have a chronic illness came up. Miserandino, who lives with lupus, used what was right in front of her and compared having lupus with having a limited collection of spoons. Living with a chronic illness means you have to "make choices or to consciously think about things when the rest of the world doesn't have to."[125]

It works like this. You get up in the morning with a certain amount of energy represented by a number of spoons (Miserandino used 12). Everything you do throughout the day takes away one or more spoons. The goal is to manage your "spoon expenditure" so that by the end of the day, you haven't used more than your daily allotment. Using more spoons than you have means you'll have to borrow from tomorrow's store, which in turn means you'll start the next day with fewer spoons available.

Some people use the analogy of spoons, others a field of lit and dark light bulbs or a bank account with the energy overdraft in red. Regardless of the image that makes sense to you, visualizing your energy as something tangible that can be measured can be very helpful. It can make it easier to accept the changes in your energy levels, can help you spend the energy more wisely and is a terrific tool to explain your reality to others.

Which brings us to the idea of pacing yourself. Sure, you've wrapped your head around the fact that you have less energy and need to be careful using it, but what does this actually look like?

Think of it this way: you need to have a **PLAN**. That means have a **P**lan B, **L**earn to say no, set **A**ttainable goals and **N**ap.

Plan B

Most people have a mental or written list of things they plan to get done in a particular timeframe (a day, a week and so on). It's how we organize our days and make sure that nothing gets left behind. Personally, I'm a big fan of lists — they keep me on track, and I thoroughly enjoy scratching things out when I'm done. In fact, I've been known to add something to a list after it's been done, just so I can have the pleasure of drawing a line through the item!

The downfall for many people with RA is having only one plan, with no alternatives. The list is there, things need to get done. If you're having a bad day, they still need to get done. This might have you plowing through the list regardless of how you feel. As many of us know, this can cause a flare that lasts for days. On the other hand, if you simply don't have the energy, having only one option can send you into hiding on the couch, feeling like a failure.

There is another option. Instead of approaching your list in an either/or manner, divide it into items that need more or less time and energy. This gives you flexibility to adjust your activity level depending on your pain and energy levels. If you have a bad day, pick a less intense task. For instance, paying your bills while seated at a desk takes less energy than vacuuming the living room. Heat up leftovers or a prepared meal from your supermarket's freezer instead of cooking from scratch. If you had plans to go out with a friend, invite them over to watch a DVD instead. And so on.

Having a Plan B (and C, D and possibly E) means you have the option of still doing something, whether your goal is to be productive or to enjoy yourself. You have now created a situation that builds successes instead of failures. This will help you feel better about yourself, which makes it easier to live with RA.

Learn to Say No

Such a little word, so very hard to say. We want to help others, want to achieve, want to be polite and most of us aren't taught to say no gracefully. Instead, we instinctively say yes, only later realizing that we have just bought ourselves a ticket on the exhaustion train. Sound familiar?

This is my Achilles heel. I have an almost pathological inability to say no, especially when something sounds interesting. In the moment, gripped by excitement or a desire to get something done quickly, I forget to think about what else is going on in my life. Soon afterwards, I've worked myself into a flare and then nothing gets done at all.

It took years of overcommitting before I learned that I have to trick myself. When people ask if I can do something, I say I'll have to check my schedule and get back to them. I usually know my schedule, but it gives me time to think about whether I have the energy, if there are other things my energy should be spent on and if I actually want to do what I'm being asked to do. Giving myself time to think means connecting to what I truly want to do and to the reality of my physical health. Knowing I have a solid reason to say no makes it easier for the word to come out of my mouth. Most of the time, anyway. I still tend to say yes more often than I should, but I'm getting better at recognizing my limits.

My trick might work for you, as well, or maybe something else would be more helpful. Spend some time thinking about what happens when you say yes and later think you shouldn't have. Think about why you said yes and how quickly you realized it might have been a bad idea. Analyzing these types of situations and your own reactions and feelings connected to them will help you identify a strategy to protect your energy and reduce your pain.

Attainable Goals

Everyone I know has a tendency to overestimate how much they can do. When you're healthy, overdoing it can lead to an exhausted weekend. When you have RA, it can trigger a domino effect that can seriously interfere with your life. Doing too much can lead to severe fatigue and even a flare, increasing swelling and pain. Recovering from a flare can mean sitting on the couch for several days or longer, sometimes even having to get a booster pack of prednisone from your doctor.

To avoid this domino effect it's better to *underestimate* how much you can do. When you set yourself a goal, make sure it's attainable, something you know you can easily do. This has several benefits in addition to preventing a flare. Attainable goals can help you build on success, making you feel better about yourself. In the long run, you'll get more done.

As an example, let's consider my dining room table, aka the horizontal filing area. Because I use a wheelchair and have some serious mobility issues, I tend to use my dining room table as a temporary storage area. Cleaning up bores me, and I only have so much energy, which I tend to use on other things. As you can imagine, my dining room table is often a bit of a mess. When the files take over, I'll set myself a goal of dealing with three pieces of paper every day. When those three pieces of paper are done, I'll walk away. Using this method means I won't have to take long breaks while I nurse a flare caused by doing it all in one day. As well, I can also do the other things in my life that require my attention, such as work, buying groceries and so on. My three pieces of paper a day leads to a clean table faster than you'd think, and I keep my pain levels manageable. Setting attainable goals taught me that slow and steady really does win the race.

Another example is exercise. Getting in shape can help you stay flexible and keep your muscles strong, which supports your joints. Some people who have well-controlled RA are able to exercise at the same level as those who do not have the disease. However, others who have a more active disease or are very much in touch with their inner couch potato may have more of a challenge to get fit. Unless you're an athlete, deciding you want to exercise every day is likely to set you up for failure. Life gets in the way, you're too tired or you hurt too much. Before you know it, you're busy beating yourself up because you haven't met your goal. On the other hand, setting a goal of exercising twice a week is more easily attainable (unless you're flat on your back with a flare, of course). This creates a success, which makes you feel good about yourself.

Setting attainable goals can be used for pretty much everything: gardening, cleaning up the house, learning to meditate (see Chapter 35), organizing the garage, dealing with a pile of mail — you get the idea. Setting a goal that seems ridiculously easy might seem, well, ridiculous at first. After all, anyone can do three pieces of paper every day, right? Setting an easy goal ensures that you'll be able to do a little every time you do the task in question. Building success upon success makes you feel much better about yourself and your ability to meet your goals. And in the long run it often gets a lot more done.

Nap

As I mentioned at the start of this chapter, RA often comes hand in hand with a significant amount of fatigue. This can mean that people with RA need more sleep than others do, often "over 10 hours of sleep a night, or eight hours a night and a two-hour nap during the day."[126] That's a lot of sleep.

You may be able to manage the extra hours of sleep by going to bed earlier, but napping can be a bit more difficult to arrange. Most of us would love to have a siesta in the middle of the day, but resist. Adults don't, do they? Adults have more important things to do than indulging themselves with the luxury of a nap.

Not so fast. When you have RA, a nap may not be indulgent. It can be one of the most important things you do.

Several years ago, it became necessary for me to have a nap every afternoon to manage my pain and energy. Without that rest in the middle of the day, I'd run out of energy (or spoons), and my pain levels would go through the roof. With the nap, I have the energy I need to get through my day and, most of the time, pain that is easier to manage. To shut people up who remarked on how lovely it must be to be able to nap — thereby inferring that I have nothing better to do — and to emphasize the necessity of the rest, I changed the language I used. I stopped using the word "nap" and instead now call it my Mandatory Rest Period.

Admittedly, I am a writer who only shares her apartment with a silly cat. Both of these factors make it easier for me to adjust my schedule to incorporate a nap. When you work outside of the home and have children, finding time to have a Mandatory Rest Period can seem almost impossible. Thinking creatively may help you find an opportunity. Does your employer have a sick room that you can use? Could your spouse mind the children for half an hour when you get home? Can you lie down on the couch while the kids do their homework?

Lying down, even for half an hour, can do wonders for your ability to do what you need to do. If your body tells you that you need to take a rest, listen to it. Make an appointment with YOU, tuck yourself in with a warm blanket and let your body regenerate. This helps you to regain a spoon or two that you'll need for the rest of the day. If the people in your life don't understand the importance of what you're doing, call the naps Mandatory Rest Periods instead.

Learning to pace yourself takes time. It means putting your own needs first, something we often instinctively label as "selfish" and therefore undesirable. It isn't. As with so many other preconceived notions, it helps to turn it around and look at it another way. More specifically, think of what I call "The Yellow Oxygen Mask Rule."

When you fly, the flight attendants will take you through the safety procedures. Should the cabin pressure change, the yellow oxygen masks will fall from the ceiling. If you are flying with a child or someone else who is dependent on you, you must apply the mask to yourself first. It sounds selfish, but there is a very good reason for this. If you are responsible for someone else, you must stay conscious. If you first put the mask on the person you are taking care of, you may pass out and therefore be absolutely no help to them.

Your energy is your oxygen, whether you have RA or not. Without energy, you can't help other people. Taking care of yourself actually enables you to be a better employee, son or daughter, spouse, parent and friend. When you have RA, taking care of yourself is even more important. Meeting your need for more sleep and rest protects your store of spoons. The more spoons you have, the more helpful you can be to others and the better you'll feel physically. Implementing the **PLAN** in your life will help you feel better, and the people who need you will benefit.

37

Filters, Focus and Fun

"I was fine a minute ago..."

You've been out with friends, doing what you love best — sitting around a table debating the mysteries of life, tapping your toes to good music, eating a great meal — and you can't remember the last time you laughed that much. You feel fantastic, but when you get home and close the front door behind you, there's an almost immediate rush of exhaustion and pain. The thought of lifting a toothbrush makes you want to cry, so you go to bed with some painkillers and slightly fuzzy teeth. What's going on?

It's the Fun Filter and it's one of the most effective painkillers around.

You learn to live with pain. You learn to filter out the cranky bitching from various parts of your body, so what comes through is not quite as loud as it could be. Don't believe me? Try it sometime. Take a routine task that doesn't require a lot of focus and that you normally don't associate with pain. Depending on the severity of your RA, it can range from making a cup of tea to folding the laundry or picking up your toddler's toys. When you do, pay a lot of attention to what you're doing and what it feels like. Unless you're in remission, you'll probably discover that some of these routine tasks are accompanied by more pain than you normally think they are.

Filters happen when you shift your focus. When you first begin to live with the pain of RA, it can seem all-consuming, as if there is nothing else in your life but this overwhelming sensation. It's almost impossible to see or feel anything else — your focus is on what is happening within your body. As time goes on and you find a medication that manages your disease and another medication that reduces the pain — and even if you don't — you begin to focus outward again. That's when the filters start to develop.

Our minds are wonderfully one-track organisms. We live in a world so busy that multitasking has become the new normal, but there is increasing evidence that it actually reduces your performance. We can multitask in certain contexts — for instance, walking and talking — but our brains are "biologically incapable of processing attention-rich inputs simultaneously."[127] In other words, if you started paying attention to the minute details of walking, your ability to hold a coherent conversation would go downhill very quickly.

You can use this knowledge of your one-track mind to reduce your experience of pain. Immersing yourself in activities you enjoy or that challenge you mentally shifts your focus and can therefore block a significant amount of your pain. On the really bad days, it can be as simple as what type of relatively passive entertainment you choose. Lying wrapped up in a blanket on the couch doing nothing will make you feel more of your pain than if you're wrapped up in a blanket on the couch watching a movie or reading a good book. On better days, finding something more challenging can absorb more of your focus. Writing poetry, drawing, doing crosswords or Sudoku, taking photographs, gardening, having a rousing debate about politics or doing something that makes you laugh can all help shift your focus. It doesn't matter if your poetry is horrible, you can only draw stick figures or your photographs are always slightly askew. What matters is finding an activity that captivates your interest and engages your mind.

This one-track approach isn't just mental, it works for your body, too. Someone once told me that your nerves can only interpret one thing at a time. It's why the pain of contractions during labor can be eased by pouring water over the woman's stomach. Using another stimulus or sensation confuses the nerves and reduces the experience of pain. I once shared this interesting factoid with my partner and, smart man that he is, he extrapolated and regularly uses it to help me. When I'm in a lot of pain, he'll hold my hand, caressing my skin with his thumb, or run his fingers through my hair. In these small ways, he reminds my nerve endings that they aren't only made for relaying the sensation of pain.

Other ways of distracting your nerve endings include stroking your dog or cat and knitting or crocheting if you can — it keeps your fingers mobile and the sensual pleasure of soft yarn sliding through your fingers is a great distraction. You can also place aching joints under running water or sit in the sun with the wind in your hair. Experiment and play around. You'll find ways that work for you.

Be it mental or physical — or both at the same time — distraction can be an important tool to reduce your experience of pain. Finding ways of developing filters can help turn down the volume on your pain several notches. You may have started out with your pain at a level seven on a ten-point scale, but doing something creative reduces your experience of the pain to a five. On a really bad day with very high pain levels, disappearing into a good movie or book can help reduce your pain to something tolerable. And on good days, focusing on something you enjoy or that challenges your mind can make you feel almost pain-free.

One warning, though: check in with your body every now and again to see how it's doing. I have a stubborn habit of getting lost in various activities on my computer, such as writing or editing photographs. When I do, it filters out the pain so efficiently that I only hear my body's messages when it's begging for mercy. That's why writing many of the chapters in this book were quickly followed by me having to take big painkillers. I'm happy to report that the lesson started to stick around the time I wrote the Pain Management section, and I now have a habit of doing the "body check" at around the 400-word mark. Most of the time.

38
Surgery

"I have become the bionic woman!"

Between the beginning of summer and Christmas in my sixteenth year, I had both hips replaced. My hips had fused when I was fourteen, making it impossible for me to sit. I'd spent two years lying in a hospital bed while I waited for my bionic parts. This was in Denmark in the late 1970s, and replacement joints came from England. It could take a while, especially when you needed the spare parts custom-made because the regular sizes wouldn't fit your bones. I still remember my surprise when after the surgery-related pain abated, not only could I move my hips again, but they didn't hurt anymore! Five weeks after the second hip was replaced, I got a power wheelchair and, after years living in hospitals, this was when my life started again. I went back to school, made friends, participated in gatherings of my extended family, talked on the phone and everything else that comes with a regular teenage life.

Surgery — often lots of it — used to be inevitable for people with RA. For so long, there were hardly any treatments, so progression of the disease would lead to the kind of damage that required surgery in order to reduce pain and delay disability. These days, the likelihood of someone with RA needing surgery has decreased significantly.[128] We now have many more medication options to treat RA and to treat it more effectively than when I was a child. Because of these meds, people who have RA now generally have less destructive joint damage than in the past. This means fewer surgeries overall.

Unfortunately, not all of us respond to medication, and joint damage still happens. If it has a pronounced impact on your function and quality of life, surgery can help reduce pain and increase mobility. It's still a big step, and most doctors do their best to delay surgery for as long as possible. Other types of treatment and techniques may be used to try to resolve the problem, such as physical therapy (see Chapter 39), splints and braces and occupational therapy (see Chapter 40).

If other techniques don't resolve the problem, your rheumatologist may recommend surgery. They will refer you to an orthopedic surgeon, a doctor who specializes in conditions involving muscles and bones. Orthopedic surgeons perform a variety of procedures for people who have RA. Some of these surgeries are for soft tissues and some are for the joints.

Common surgeries for RA include:

Synovectomy

This type of surgery removes the synovium (the tissue lining the joint), thereby reducing inflammation and preventing joint damage. A synovectomy is usually done earlier in the disease progression when there is minimal joint damage. It can be done using arthroscopy, a type of surgery in which procedures are done through a thin tube inserted into a joint through a small slit in the skin.[129] This minimizes scarring and usually requires less recovery time. A synovectomy is a more temporary solution and inflammation may return.[130]

Tendon Repair

RA inflammation doesn't just happen in the joints, it also affect tendons. Severe swelling can cause tendons to rupture or split, which leads to loss of function. The tendons in the hands are particularly vulnerable and, if they're damaged, you may not be able to use your fingers.

Two types of tendons are most commonly affected in RA. Extensor tendons run across the back of the hand. Damage in these tendons can lead to being unable to straighten one or more fingers. Flexor tendons run along the wrist and palm. Flexor tendon damage may mean that you are unable to make a fist, use your fingers or grip an object.[131]

In such cases, the orthopedic surgeon will do a procedure called a tendon repair, essentially stitching the damaged tendon back together.[132] Flexor tendon repair is the more complicated procedure of the two, because it is more difficult to get to and near a number of important nerves.

Carpal Tunnel Release

You have probably heard of carpal tunnel syndrome before. It can happen with repetitive strain injuries, particularly in people who use their hands a lot, such as those with jobs that require a lot of typing.

The carpal tunnel is located in your forearm, just before your wrist. It's a narrow tunnel containing ligaments, bone and the median nerve. Conditions that cause swelling or change of position in the tissue of that area can irritate and compress the median nerve. When that happens, you experience tingling and numbness of the thumb, index and middle fingers.[133] This can affect your ability to use your hands to grip. When you have RA, swelling and inflammation can compress the carpal tunnel and affect your median nerve.

Carpal tunnel release is the name of the surgery used to correct carpal tunnel syndrome. In this procedure, the surgeon cuts the carpal ligament to reduce pressure on the nerve.[134]

Joint Fusion

The damage of active RA can cause a joint to become unstable or misaligned. If joint replacement is not an option, the surgeon may recommend that you have the joint fused (also called arthrodesis). Fusing a joint makes it immobile, which means it is more stable, can more easily bear weight and is no longer painful.[135]

In this surgery, bones are held against each other with screws until they grow together and become rigid. This kind of surgery is more common in smaller joints like fingers and toes, as well as ankles, wrists and the spine.[136]

Fusing a joint sounds really drastic and sort of counterintuitive — how can immobilizing the joint lead to better function? No longer being in pain is a big help, and misaligned or unstable joints can be very difficult to use. I happen to be one of the people for whom RA largely fuses joints, rather than rendering them unstable. Most of this damage happened by the time I was in my late teens, and I can tell you from firsthand experience that you adapt very quickly. The stability and lack of pain more than offset any loss of mobility.

Joint Replacement

Total joint replacement is a last resort when a joint has been damaged so severely that other treatments cannot address the loss of function and/or high pain levels. The problems caused by an extremely damaged joint are likely to cause you to avoid using it as much as possible. When that happens, your muscles may atrophy and weaken, leading to more loss of function.

Replacements of larger joints like hips and knees have been quite common for several decades and are usually very successful. People with RA may also have their shoulders and elbows replaced. Replacement of a smaller joint, such as a finger, is a more recently developed procedure and can be trickier.

In joint replacement procedures, the surgeon will remove the damaged bone and replace it with a prosthetic joint made of metal, plastic or a combination of both. For instance, if you have a hip replacement, the upper part of your femur (thighbone) is removed and a prosthetic hip joint (the ball at the top of the femur) inserted into the bone. A cup is then placed in the pelvis bone, and the ball is connected to the cup, just like the connection in a healthy hip joint.

A joint replacement will not restore complete function in your joint, but to someone who's lived with severe pain and limited mobility for a long time, it can seem close enough to qualify as a miracle.

Risks and Benefits of Surgery

Surgery is an intense procedure. Being under general anesthetic, cut open and manipulated in various ways is pretty serious stuff. Surgery of any kind does carry some risks, primarily related to the general anesthetic, bleeding and possible infection.

There are a number of different ways to mitigate the risk. Some surgeons recommend that you donate your own blood before the surgery because it is easier for your body to deal with. It also cuts down the risk of receiving contaminated blood, although these days, there are very good safeguards in place for donated blood. Prior to your surgery, your doctor will meet with you to discuss what will happen during and after the surgery. You'll also sign a consent form. This is one of those moments when the notion of informed consent can seem a little scary, but knowing what you're facing will make the recovery easier.

There are things you can do to cut down the risks and improve your experience of surgery and recovery. The first is to find a good surgeon, and your rheumatologist will be able to help you with that. Another way to prepare yourself is to research the procedure and come prepared to your appointment with the surgeon with a list of questions. These include your surgeon's background and experience, success rates of that particular surgery, pros and cons of doing the procedure and so on. You may also want to research surgery in general and what to expect during your hospital stay.

The benefits of surgery are quite obvious to people who live with RA. Less pain — or no pain at all — and increased mobility. Be aware that the recovery and rehabilitation period can take a while. In the long run, though, most people end up better than they were before.

Recovery and Rehab

There are two stages to recovery from surgery. The first is what happens between you waking up in the recovery room and going home, which will be later that day or several days after the surgery, depending on the procedure. Two things are pretty common when you wake up after surgery: nausea and pain. There's something about the general anesthetic that pokes at a lot of people's stomachs. It's a good idea to talk to your surgeon or anesthesiologist about ways to reduce the potential for nausea. Sometimes different types of anesthetics can help reduce the likelihood of nausea. If you are nauseated after you wake up, there are other medications that can help, as well. You'll have an IV of saline solution as you go in to surgery, to ensure you stay hydrated. Most people don't eat or drink a lot after surgery, so the IV may stay in your arm for a couple of days. If you're nauseated after surgery, the doctor may order anti-nausea drugs for the IV.

There will be pain after the surgery, and for the first couple of days, it can be quite intense. It is different than RA pain — sharper, somehow cleaner — and one of the best things about post-surgery pain is that it gets a little bit better every day.

Another good thing about post-surgery pain is that you won't be expected to get through it on your own. When you first wake up, you may receive pain medication through your IV or in a shot. If you've had day surgery, you'll get a prescription for opioids to manage the pain when you go home. If you have a larger surgery, such as a hip replacement, you'll stay in the hospital for several days. For the first two to three days after the surgery, you will probably receive pain medication through an IV, usually in the form of a morphine pump where you press a button to receive pain relief when you need it. Around the third day, you'll switch to painkillers in tablet form, but they will still be opioids. When you get discharged from the hospital, you'll go home with a prescription for painkillers, likely some form of opioids, as well. Take them. No one expects you to get back on your feet without them. In fact, your recovery will likely be better if you have good pain control.

The second stage of recovery relates to building up strength and mobility again. This will start very quickly after your surgery, with nursing staff getting you out of bed and moving around. A physical therapist will also get involved fairly soon after your surgery. As well, some kinds of surgery will require you to immobilize the part of your body that was operated on until the healing process is complete. For instance, a joint fusion will typically require a cast or brace for a few months to keep the joint still while the bone fuses over the metal screws and pins.

When you're ready, a physical therapist will help you put together a more intense exercise program that can make you stronger and improve your mobility. Rehab is hard work and can be tiring and at times painful. Again, make sure you take your painkillers as prescribed to help you to be able to do the work. The rehab experience is very different than the fatigue and pain that comes with RA. As you do your exercises, you'll notice an improvement. This gives you a goal to work towards and can be a very positive experience. Keep going. The results will be worth it.

Depending on the surgery, it can take two to three months before you are healed and well enough to get back in the swing of things. Be patient with yourself during this time. Your body has been through a lot, and it's going to take a while for it to return to normal. Give yourself the rest and understanding you need in order to make the surgery a success.

The medications available today mean that surgery isn't as common in the treatment of RA as it used to be. However, people who have had RA for years, or who don't respond well to current medications and other treatments, are still at risk for significant joint damage. For those individuals, surgery can play an important role in decreasing pain and improving function. Having an operation is an intense experience, but making yourself aware of what will happen before you go into the hospital will make recovery easier. Some people get nervous at the thought of surgery, but if you live with the kind of problems that warrant an operation, you already have the skills needed to get through the experience. Best of all, recovery from surgery is time-limited and at the end, your ability to live your life will have improved.

39

Physical Therapy

"How am I supposed to exercise when I hurt this much?"

Physical therapy has been part of my life since I was a child. My first memory of doing exercises prescribed to me by a physical therapist was after surgery. When I was ten years old, I had a synovectomy on my right wrist to deal with the inflammation and pain that was limiting me in my daily life. Afterwards, I did exercises every day to increase the mobility in my wrist. I remember sitting at the dining room table, putting my hand flat on its surface and lifting my elbow, bending the wrist as far as it could go. Since that time, I have seen numerous physical therapists and have done pretty much every kind of exercise and activity they have for RA. My favorite was always exercises in a heated pool. The buoyancy of the water took the stress off my joints, making it possible to just enjoy moving without pain.

Physical therapy is a discipline within the field of rehabilitation medicine. The goal of treatment is to "restore, maintain and maximize your strength, function, movement and overall well-being."[137] What you call it depends on what country you live in — physical therapy in the US, physiotherapy in Canada, the UK and Australia. No matter what you call it, it's an essential tool for managing RA.

A physical therapist is an accredited health professional with a graduate degree, licensed to practice in a particular state or province. They are trained to assess and treat symptoms of various illnesses and conditions that affect how you move. Examples include rehab after an injury such as a broken leg, building up strength after a long illness and helping people with chronic illnesses control pain and maintain their level of function.

Being physically active is important for people who live with RA. The old adage "use it or lose it" applies especially to the various kinds of arthritis. If you don't move, your joints may stiffen up and fuse, affecting your mobility in the future. Being active will also help you stay as fit as possible, which is important for your general health and the health of your joints. Following an exercise program can help you develop muscle tone to support your joints, making you stronger and reducing pain. It's important to make sure that you move in a smart way that builds ability, rather than putting undue strain on joints. This is where physical therapy enters the picture.

A physical therapist is your partner in getting to a place of strength and well-being. They do this by tailoring exercises and treatment to your specific needs. Their approach is comprehensive, including factors in your life that may affect how you feel, whether you're in pain and which joints need extra care. Recommendations for someone who is in remission or who has mild RA are going to be very different from the suggestions given to someone who has a more severe form of the disease.

Physical therapists don't just treat you with exercises and strengthening activities. They also provide you with education about how your body moves and how to move better. This can help you build strength and mobility and reduce pain and injury. As well, your therapist can connect you to services in your community that may be of use in staying physically active, helping with aspects of daily living and so on, such as aqua fit programs, home care and others.

A number of different exercises may be used for people living with RA:

Range of motion (ROM) moves each individual joint through its full range and helps to reduce pain and stiffness. This is the gentlest form of exercise and is usually safe to do even for inflamed and flaring joints.

Strengthening exercises can stabilize your joints by building strong muscles. This is usually done by traditional strengthening activities involving resistance. Be aware that resistance exercises can aggravate flaring joints. If your RA is active in certain joints, be sure to mention it to your physical therapist so you can adapt the exercises as necessary.

Stretching exercises are typically done after the strengthening activity to increase flexibility in muscles and tendons. This can help reduce the risk of contractures and retain full movement of a joint.

Aerobic exercise improves the health of your heart and lungs. Which kind of aerobic exercise will work for you depends on your level of disease activity and/or damage in your joints.

Hydrotherapy (exercise in water) puts less stress on your joints, making it easier to move. As well, the buoyancy of the water provides natural resistance, which helps you build strength.[138] This kind of therapy is usually done in heated pools, which can feel wonderful for sore joints.

We are often taught that the principle of exercise is "no pain, no gain." This is not the case for those of us who have RA. It is important *not to* exercise to the point of pain, even when you're doing range of motion. If you overdo exercise, it can lead to a flare that can last for days. Work within your limits, not beyond them. Stop if it hurts. A physical therapist can teach you how to assess which kinds of exercises should be used at different levels of disease activity. This will help you know when to do particular exercises and when not to push a flaring joint.

In addition to helping you develop an exercise program that will be best for your individual case, physical therapists offer a number of treatments that can help you manage pain:

TENS (transcutaneous electrical nerve stimulation) uses electrodes placed on your skin that give a low level, safe electric stimulation of nerves. It sounds a little unsettling, but usually you only feel a mild buzzing. Some people find this kind of treatment very helpful for pain.

Ultrasound used for therapeutic purposes is different from diagnostic ultrasound that is used to get a picture of a fetus or an organ. Therapeutic ultrasound heats up soft tissue, allowing more blood and oxygen to flow through the area. It is especially helpful for issues related to muscle strain or spasms.

Massage can be helpful in treating tight muscles. It's important to be extra careful around the neck area, as this part of the spine may be affected by RA.[139] (For more details about massage, see Chapter 34.)

Acupuncture is increasingly being used by physical therapists to reduce pain. (For more, see Chapter 33.)

How to Find a Physical Therapist

It's important that your physical therapist knows your diagnosis and the issues that may affect your care. They will also need direction from your doctor in terms of the specific goals of treatment. This is why you need a referral from your rheumatologist, orthopedic surgeon or family doctor in order to access physical therapy.

Physical therapy is different for previously healthy people who are recovering from a broken leg and for those of us who have a chronic illness or live with chronic pain. Not all physical therapists have experience working with chronic conditions and I recommend that you do your best to find someone who does. Discuss the issue with the referring doctor to see if they can recommend a particular clinic or therapist to help you in your quest for better health. When you meet the physical therapist, they will start by asking about your history and current situation. They will also include a physical exam to assess your current ability to move. If something hurts, make sure you speak up. It's important that the therapist knows your boundaries — it will help them give you better treatment.

Physical therapy may be covered by your insurance or for some, by public funds. Others may have to pay for it themselves and that can be a challenge. Talk to your doctor about the possibility of finding a clinic that provides treatment based on a sliding fee schedule, where you pay according to your income. If money is tight, you can also talk to your physical therapist about ways to get the most "bang for your buck."

Keep in mind that RA affects people in different ways, and your individual case may therefore affect which kinds of exercises are safe for you to do. Talk to your rheumatologist about whether you need to be especially careful of certain joints. Once you've had that conversation, ask for a referral to a physical therapist.

Using physical therapy can be an invaluable tool for anyone with RA, helping to improve mobility and strength and reduce pain. Finding a way to be active while protecting your joints will ultimately help you live your life as fully and independently as possible.

40
Occupational Therapy

"All that stands between me and jam on my toast is the blasted lid on the jar."

When I was a child, I spent a lot of time in a rehab hospital. Being away from home for months at a time was hard, but I always looked forward to my turn in the occupational therapy department. Different kinds of therapies were used depending on your condition, but to me as a kid with juvenile rheumatoid arthritis, the therapy was more like play. I did a lot of textile printing, dipping blocks with cutout designs into paint and carefully applying them to fabric. In this way I made aprons for my mother, a tablecloth for my grandmother and stuffed animals for my little sister. I made pendants out of coconut shells, sanding off the rough parts, leaving a beautiful deep brown surface. Every now and again, I baked cookies.

Occupational therapy, like physical therapy (see Chapter 39), is a discipline within the field of rehabilitation medicine. Occupational therapists (OTs) are specialists in assessing a person's level of function to identify ways to improve that function. They help people "participate in the things they want and need to do through the therapeutic use of everyday activities."[140] This is what happened at the rehab hospital when I was a child. The occupational therapists kept my hands and fingers mobile by engaging me in activities that used dexterity and strength. This was a vital part of ensuring that my joints could function and helped me be as independent as possible. There was a direct link between the fun activities I was doing and my ability to, for instance, button a shirt.

Occupational therapists help you improve function through a variety of treatments, techniques and tools. One such treatment is the use of splints. Made of hard material, splints are used to provide support to or immobilize a part of your body. One common use of this technique is wrapping a broken bone in a cast, immobilizing it until it knits back together. A cast is wrapped around the affected part of your body and you cannot take it off. Splints, on the other hand, are more like a half cast held in place by an elastic bandage or Velcro straps and can be easily adjusted or removed.

Two types of splints are typically used to treat RA. The first kind helps increase the joint's range of motion by progressively straightening it so it doesn't become fixed or fused in one place. The second kind of splint is designed to hold the joint in one particular position, allowing the joint and muscles to rest.[141] Splints can be a very helpful tool in reducing pain. By supporting and stabilizing a joint, for instance a wrist, a splint can keep a flare from increasing when you use your hand. As well, keeping your wrist immobile and supported can increase your ability to function in your everyday routine.[142]

Function is a key concept in occupational therapy. The goal is to enable you to do what you need and want to do throughout your day, whether it is at home or at work. If you have problems doing what are called tasks of daily living — such as dealing with buttons, zippers, kitchen tools and so on — an OT can help you be more independent. They can also be helpful at your workplace, making it easier for you to do the tasks of your job.

You can be coping exceptionally well with your diagnosis, moving on with your life, keeping it together and showing poise and composure at all times. And then you can't open the pickle jar and you fall apart.

Opening jars is a breaking point for many. It's such a little thing and yet so hugely symbolic of the impact RA can have on your life. You don't know what's worse: not being able to open the jar yourself or having to ask your eight-year-old to do it for you. This is where an occupational therapist can be a lifesaver.

An OT can come into your home and talk to you about your daily activities and what is difficult for you to do. After this discussion, they'll usually get out a big catalog with pages and pages of adaptive equipment, also called aids for daily living. It could be as simple as a piece of thick, sticky material that can keep a bowl steady or help you get a good grip on the lid of a jar. Knives with the handle placed at a 90° angle make it possible to cut without bending your wrist. Triangular rubber grips can be placed on pens and pencils to make writing more comfortable for aching fingers. Other types of assistance include tips and tricks for easier ways to get through your day. Examples include putting a stool in the kitchen so you can sit while you're cutting vegetables, better ways of carrying your purse and tips on energy management.

Consulting an occupational therapist can be a very surprising experience — most people have no idea how many helpful tools are out there. Even if you don't feel you're having much trouble, an OT can be very useful. They may be able to identify areas where certain tools or techniques can help reduce the strain on your body and energy. This can make it easier for you to do the things you need to do around the house and reduce pain as you go about your day. Before you know it, you're back to living your life instead of worrying about details such as opening the pickle jar.

Unless you work in a deli or restaurant, you're not likely to encounter a pickle jar at your place of employment, but the same principle applies. There may be tasks that are difficult for you to do physically, and an occupational therapist can help you find workarounds or tools to do your job so you don't have to worry about details.

At work, consulting an occupational therapist usually involves an ergonomic assessment. Ergonomics is defined as "the science of designing a person's environment so that it facilitates the highest level of function."[143] Many companies are aware that ergonomic assessments will help prevent injuries and therefore increase productivity. As well, such assessments can be part of the process when an injured employee returns to work.

This kind of assessment can include taking a look at your job description and the tasks you perform as part of your work. By assessing the tasks and your physical needs and ability, the OT can identify areas where changes can be made to help you work better. This can include modifying equipment to make it easier on your body.

An occupational therapist may also recommend accommodations. This means modifications to make the process or tasks of a job accessible to ensure that your employer complies with the Americans with Disabilities Act (ADA). In Canada, accommodation of disability is required under human rights law, such as provincial Human Rights Codes.

Many people with chronic illnesses don't realize that the ADA or human rights legislation also apply to them. They do. And if you need them, they can be a very valuable support for you to maintain your ability to work. Because of these types of legislation, your employer is legally obligated to find reasonable accommodations for you, making the job physically easier to do. Through this process, it may be possible for you to keep your job and for your employer to keep a happy and productive worker.

There are times when it may not be feasible to accommodate you. The key is whether the way in which you do your job can be reworked so that you can reach the goal of a particular task. For instance, I use a wheelchair due to severe RA and have limited ability and strength. This means that I cannot be accommodated in becoming a firefighter. However, I can probably be accommodated in many types of office work. In cases where it is not possible to adapt your job, an occupational therapist may be able to help find you another type of work within the same organization.

If you go home from work every day feeling exhausted and sore, or certain tasks are difficult for you to do, consider asking your employer for an ergonomic assessment. The process of accommodation is often fairly easy and inexpensive, but you do need an expert. You and your supervisor may not be able to figure out ways of adapting the tasks, and it can make your worry about losing your job. A consultation with an OT may make a huge difference in your ability to do your work without pain. This will make you a more productive employee who'll likely need less sick time, and that will make both you and your boss happy!

How to Find an Occupational Therapist

When you talk to your family doctor or rheumatologist about getting a referral to an occupational therapist, they will usually be able to recommend a specific clinic, agency or therapist for you. Although you can contact an OT without a referral, it may help in covering the cost. If you have health insurance, find out if this kind of service is covered and whether it's necessary to get a referral from your doctor.

You can also look for an OT yourself by contacting the professional occupational therapist association in your country. In the US, you can search on the website of the American Occupational Therapy Association, Inc. (www.aota.org). In Canada, the Canadian Association of Occupational Therapists also has a search function on their website (www.caot.ca). In other areas, use your favorite search engine and type "occupational therapist" and the name of your country.

So much of the frustration of having RA is related to its impact on the tasks that you do every day. You may be able to wrap your head around having a chronic illness and taking medication that suppresses your immune system. And then you come up against something that you used to do with ease, and the reality hits you hard. RA can impact many of the tasks in your home and at work, making them harder to do and causing you pain or worries. Talking to an occupational therapist can be an important step in finding ways to function better and be more independent. Not having to rely on your children to open a jar can do wonders for your emotional health. Finding ways for your work not to wreck you physically will help you feel more secure in your job and make you more productive. When things are easier to do both at home and at work, you'll feel more like yourself again. Once you do that, you can get back to focusing on living.

41

Pain Management Wrap-Up

"Couldn't you just hit me over the head with a two-by-four?"

When you first experience the kind of pain that can come with uncontrolled RA, it can be scary, overwhelming and leave you emotionally curled up in a ball. This is normal. If you've never had unmanageable or high levels of pain, it can make you feel quite desperate and depressed. It can make you worry that you're doomed to live in constant pain.

The advances made in creating new medications have had a drastic effect on how RA is treated. The approach is now to treat early and aggressively, and it's working for many more people than ever before. Some have little or no pain. Some only have pain when they really push themselves. Some have moderate pain levels on and off, some have chronic pain and sometimes, it's both severe and chronic. I am convinced that in the future there will be fewer and fewer people with RA who have severe or chronic pain. At this point in time, however, whether it is from inflammation or damaged joints (or both), many of us live in a reality that includes some level of pain.

And this is where I'm about to get a bit revolutionary.

Pain isn't the worst thing that can happen.

People tend to look at me funny when I say that. Pain is bad, isn't it? It isn't normal to have pain. Pain makes you cry, makes it hard to move and prevents you from doing things.

Doesn't it?

I have lived with chronic pain since I was four years old, and it has taught me a different perspective. I have learned that even without RA, pain is part of life. Whether it is stubbing your toe, the ache that comes with an excellent workout or the loss of a loved one, there's no avoiding it.

The good news is that the power of adapting to change seems to be hardwired in the human psyche. That comes in very handy when you live with pain.

Having had chronic pain for over four decades has taught me that the question isn't pain or no pain. The question is whether the pain is taking over your life or is something that can be managed well enough that you can get on with things. This philosophy applies both to heartbreak and physical pain. And this is where that ability to adapt really kicks in. The goal becomes managing the pain so it subsides enough that you can focus on other things.

If you're relatively new at this, you may still be looking at me funny, doubting that this can be possible. Trust me. It is. You learn to use tools to lower the pain and to decrease your experience of it. Sometimes you use external tools such as medication, heat or ice, and time will tell you what works best in which combination. Sometimes more internal tools such as managing your energy or meditation can teach you to change the way you live your life and thereby have an impact on your pain levels. Through it all, the natural human ability to adapt will gradually help you develop filters that change your experience of the pain.

Learning the tricks to manage your RA pain comes with time. You can help the process along by staying committed to living your life as fully as possible. When you put your life first, it creates an expectation within you that achieving manageable pain is possible. This helps you pursue solutions from a position of empowerment. And best of all, it means you're out there, living your life regardless of the pain.

42
Living Your Life with RA

When you live with RA there are days when it will suck to be you. Sometimes, it will be because a flare is making you feel as if you're dragging around a dead weight while someone's trying to pry apart your joints with a knife.[144] At other times, it will be a visit of the "if onlys," wishing fervently you didn't have the limits RA has forced upon you. And then there's having to take medication for the rest of your life. Separately or all at once, some days these things will hit you, and you'll take a swim in the self-pity pool. Don't let anyone tell you that this isn't OK. When you live in a situation that is objectively and realistically Not Fun, it's all right to be upset about it at times. The trick is not making the self-pity a lifestyle.

I call it "Having a Swish." It means doing your best not to wallow in the self-pity pool. Every now and again, though, when it feels like you're fighting for your life — usually metaphorically — you swish your feet around in the self-pity pool for a little while. And then you climb out, snarl in the face of the disease, refuse to give up and refuse to be defined by it.

It's not always easy, this fighting for your life, but it is an essential aspect of finding part of every day that belongs to you alone. Something that represents your life, enabling you to live with RA, but not be controlled by it. It is a delicate balance, fueled by that snarling refusal to relinquish control, expressed through hope, optimism and the quest for joy. This is what will get you through. This is what will help you stay true to who you are, what will keep you from all-encompassing despair. It is turning the prism through which you see your life and looking through a different facet, one that emphasizes the positive.

What helps you see this? It starts with accepting that having RA can be part of a good life. With knowing that there are things in this world that are worse than the difficulties that come with having a chronic illness.

That no longer living your life to the best of your ability is much, much worse. It includes monitoring yourself to make sure you don't get stuck in a place where you accept unreasonable symptoms. It means seeing your doctor for help to control your RA, your pain or the depression that can accompany times of struggle. Not giving up does not mean soldiering through on your own. It means not giving up the faith, the knowledge that there is a solution to your problem and that together, you and your medical team will find it.

Hope. Emily Dickinson called it "the thing with feathers,"[145] and it is what allows you to spread your wings and fly. Nourish the hope within you, look forward, never back, and every day, practice seeing the beauty and joy in life. It is all around you — in the smile on a loved one's face, in sunlight filtering through green leaves, in the taste of a ripe peach or really good chocolate. And it is in your eyes every time you look in the mirror and vow to go on.

You can do this. And you can do it well.

Your Life with Rheumatoid Arthritis

Acknowledgements

Writing is generally perceived as being a solitary activity. In reality, nurturing a manuscript and bringing it to term is anything but solitary. Finishing this book is a pretty exhilarating experience, one that makes me want to thank everyone I've ever known. The following deserve particular mention:

Dan Handler designed a cover that brilliantly conveyed everything about the book. His gracious patience and professionalism made the entire process completely painless and loads of fun. Holly Sawchuk took my baby and gave it a copy edit sent from heaven. She was gentle, encouraging and held my hand throughout changing my instinctive approach to grammar into something that actually followed rules. If you need a graphic designer or an editor, you couldn't find better than Dan and Holly — their contact info is on the credit page at the beginning of the book.

Stephen King calls them his "constant readers," the people you can trust to read a newly finished manuscript and treat it with care and honesty. I am a lucky woman, because I had a team of them. Laurie Kingston, writing buddy extraordinaire, whose talent, sharp eye and love made the periods of hard slog easier and a lot more fun. She's read every word of this twice and deserves a truckload of chocolate for it. Birthe Andersen, for overcoming the instincts of being my mother and gently telling me when I sucked. Janne Andersen-Biggs, for volunteering to read a draft while wrangling a full-time job and two lively and lovely children. And Trevor Tymchuk, my one-person research and resource department, whose attention to detail saved me on countless occasions.

A fantastic team of healthcare professionals kept me healthy and saved me from making a fool of myself. They deserve nothing but gratitude. I thank Louise Perlin for being a brilliant rheumatologist, whose care helped me get my life back and who read Part I, giving it far more attention than I'd expected. Jean Robison, for being the best family doctor I've ever known, for keeping me going throughout the years and for all the goofy jokes. Thanks are also due to Odessa Gill, doctor of naturopathic medicine and a good friend, who helped make the tips and tricks in Part II more comprehensive. And to Jan Carstoniu, pain specialist, for his input on treatment agreements and meditation and the conversations that stretched the boundaries of my mind. Any remaining errors in the book are mine.

Becoming a writer is a growth process, encouraged and nourished by a community. I want to thank Leslie Lafayette for being my mentor and Barbara McClure for taking a chance on an unknown writer all those years ago. Thanks to Joy Buchanan who hired me for HealthCentral and made me a better writer. To Allison Tsai, for being a fantastic producer and sounding board and for having my back when things get "interesting." And to the RA online community, who move and inspire me every day. I am humbled and grateful to be part of their lives.

Then there are the people without whom the act of writing would not happen. Thank you to Ken Allen for solving my technological problems for more than a decade, often before I knew I had them. Without him, I might not be a writer. And speaking of technology, to Nuance, the makers of Dragon NaturallySpeaking, without whom writing would be impossible. They don't know who I am, but without them, I'd be sitting in a corner, bored out of my mind and just getting through the day. To Abbott, for making Humira — they don't know me either, but I owe my life to this drug. To the taxpayers of Ontario (I know some of them) for helping to fund the cost of the medication that makes my life possible every day. I am beyond grateful to receive this gift. To everyone at the Clarendon Foundation who enable me to live my life every day. To Holly and Andrew Allardyce, for the gift of ultrasound that made it possible to write this book in half the time it might otherwise have taken (as well as making me a much happier person throughout). And to the contributors of the Copy Editor Stash — never has a crowdfunding event been so much fun (oink!).

Some people spark ideas and keep you motivated. I need to thank Sara Nash for saying the right thing at the right time and Leslie Vandever for the wonderful butter knife analogy. Thanks also to Linda Mcaughey for asking me how the book writing was going so many times I finally wrote one, partly just to shut her up. To my uncle Poul, for his interest and encouragement and for being a stand-in for my dad, who died too soon to see me write. And to Michele Stephens, for being there in sick and sin since 1982 and for being my biggest fan (except without the hobbling).

And then there's David Govoni. For being a partner in every sense of the word. For his tireless support, for putting up with me getting obsessive and weird when deep in the writing, for holding my hand when I flailed about consumed with doubt and anxiety and for pushing me to dream bigger than I thought possible. For the editing, the formatting and the brainstorming. And for all the grapes.

Your Life with Rheumatoid Arthritis

About the Author

Lene Andersen is a writer, health and disability advocate and photographer. She has a masters degree in social work and has had rheumatoid arthritis since early childhood, accumulating over 40 years experience of living with RA and chronic pain. Lene lives in Toronto, close to the lake and shares her home with a cat and too many books.

Visit the book website and sign up for the newsletter to be the first to hear of special events, promotions and new releases at www.yourlifewithra.com. If you'd like to send Lene an email, you can reach her at lene@yourlifewithra.com.

Endnotes

Chapter 1: The Basics of Rheumatoid Arthritis

1. *MedicineNet.com*, "Rheumatoid Arthritis (RA)." http://www.medicinenet.com/rheumatoid_arthritis/article.htm (Accessed April 11, 2011)

2. Dr. Louise Perlin, personal communication.

3. Ibid.

4. *The Arthritis Society*, "Rheumatoid Arthritis." http://www.arthritis.ca/page.aspx?pid=982 (Accessed November 9, 2012)

5. Edward Keystone, "The Most Exciting Time Ever in the History of the Treatment of Rheumatoid Arthritis." *The Arthritis Society*, http://vimeo.com/50069952(Accessed November 9, 2012)

6. Ibid.

7. Dr. Louise Perlin, personal communication.

8. Edward Keystone, "The Most Exciting Time Ever in the History of the Treatment of Rheumatoid Arthritis." *The Arthritis Society*, http://vimeo.com/50069952 (Accessed November 9, 2012)

9. Ibid.

10. Lene Andersen, "The New RA Criteria: An Interview with Dr. Gillian Hawker." *HealthCentral.com*, http://www.healthcentral.com/rheumatoid-arthritis/c/80106/130058/dr (Accessed June 18, 2011)

11. Daniel Aletaha, et.al., "2010 Rheumatoid Arthritis Classification Criteria," *Arthritis & Rheumatism* 62, no. 9 (September 2010): 2569–2581.

Chapter 3: Why Take Medication for Your RA

12. S.E. Gabriel, "Why Do People with Rheumatoid Arthritis Still Die Prematurely?" *Annals of the Rheumatic Diseases* 67 (2008):iii30–iii34.

13. Dr. Louise Perlin, personal communication.

14. *American College of Rheumatology*, "Biologic Treatments for Rheumatoid Arthritis." http://www.rheumatology.org/practice/clinical/patients/medications/biologics.asp (Accessed August 14, 2011)

15. Ibid.

16. Arthur Kavanaugh, John J. Cush, Edward C. Keystone, Craig L. Leonardi, and Ronald van Vollenhoven, "Comprehensive Disease Management and RA and Its Comorbidities." *MedscapeSME*. http://cme.medscape.com/viewarticle/586195 (reg. req.) (Accessed September 7, 2010)

Chapter 4: Medications to Suppress Your RA

17. Alan K. Matsumoto, Joan Bathon, and Clifton O. Bingham III, "Rheumatoid Arthritis Treatment." *The Johns Hopkins Arthritis Center*, http://www.hopkinsarthritis.org/arthritis-info/rheumatoid-arthritis/ra-treatment/ (Accessed August 11, 2010)

18. PJW Venables, "Patient information: Rheumatoid arthritis treatment (Beyond the Basics)." *UpToDate*, http://www.uptodate.com/contents/rheumatoid-arthritis-treatment-beyond-the-basics (Accessed November 11, 2012)

19. *The Myositis Association*, "Glossary." http://www.myositis.org/learn-about-myositis/glossary (Accessed November 11, 2012)

20. Dr. Louise Perlin, personal communication.

21. Jennifer Davis, "FDA Advisory Panel Recommends Approval of New RA Drug." *Arthritis Today*, http://www.arthritistoday.org/news/tofacitinib-fda-drug-approval195.php (Accessed November 17, 2012)

Chapter 5: Medications to Manage Pain

22. Stephen L. Tilley, Thomas M. Coffman, and Beverly H. Koller, "Mixed Messages. Modulation of Inflammation and Immune Responses by Prostaglandins and Thromboxanes," *The Journal of Clinical Investigation* 108, no. 1 (July 1, 2001): 15–23. http://www.ncbi.nlm.nih.gov/pmc/articles/PMC209346/ (Accessed April 3, 2011)

23. Carol Eustice, "Cyclooxygenase: Cox-1 and Cox-2 Explained." *About.com*, http://osteoarthritis.about.com/od/osteoarthritismedications/a/cyclooxygenase.htm (Accessed December 10, 2012)

24. *MedicineNet.com*, "Nonsteroidal Anti-Inflammatory Drugs (NSAIDs)." http://www.medicinenet.com/nonsteroidal_antiinflammatory_drugs/article.htm (Accessed August 14, 2010)

25. *WiseGeek*, "How was Aspirin Invented?" http://www.wisegeek.com/how-was-aspirin-invented.htm (Accessed November 11, 2012)

26. *Canadian Cancer Society*, "Opioid Medications." http://info.cancer.ca/cce-ecc/default.aspx?cceid=5691&toc=1&Lang=E (Accessed November 11, 2012)

Chapter 6: Financial Assistance for Medical Care and Medication

27. Lisa Emrich, "A Guide to Medical Services for the Uninsured." *HealthCentral.com*, http://www.healthcentral.com/rheumatoid-arthritis/c/72218/101658/uni (Accessed August 21, 2011)

28. Karen Lee Richards, "Finding Help When You Don't Have Insurance." *HealthCentral.com*, http://www.healthcentral.com/chronic-pain/c/5949/125551/underinsured (Accessed August 31, 2011)

29. Ibid.

30. Ibid.

31. Karen Lee Richards, "Finding Help When You Don't Have Insurance." *HealthCentral.com*, http://www.healthcentral.com/chronic-pain/c/5949/125551/underinsured (Accessed August 21, 2011)

Chapter 7: How to Take the Meds

32. *NYU Langone Medical Center*, "What's up with RA: Living Today, and Looking Forward." NYU Langone Medical Center webinar, June 7, 2011.

33. C. Grigor, et al., "Effect of the treatment strategy of tight control for rheumatoid arthritis (the TICORA study): a single-blind randomised controlled trial," *Lancet* 364, no. 9430 (July 17–23, 2004): 263-269.

34. Lene Andersen, "Remission in RA: An Interview with Dr. Yusuf Yazici." *HealthCentral.com*, http://www.healthcentral.com/rheumatoid-arthritis/c/80106/146048/dr (Accessed October 30, 2011)

Chapter 8: Remission

35. Lene Andersen, "Remission in RA: An Interview with Dr. Yusuf Yazici." *HealthCentral.com*, http://www.healthcentral.com/rheumatoid-arthritis/c/80106/146048/dr (Accessed October 30, 2011)

36. Ibid.

37. Ibid.

38. Edward Keystone, "The Most Exciting Time Ever in the History of the Treatment of Rheumatoid Arthritis." *The Arthritis Society*, http://vimeo.com/50069952 (Accessed November 9, 2012)

39. *American College of Rheumatology*, "The 2011 ACR/EULAR Definitions of Remission In Rheumatoid Arthritis Clinical Trials,. http://www.rheumatology.org/practice/clinical/classification/ra/ra_remission_2011.asp (Accessed October 30, 2011)

40. Lene Andersen, "Remission in RA: An Interview with Dr. Yusuf Yazici." *HealthCentral.com*, http://www.healthcentral.com/rheumatoid-arthritis/c/80106/146048/dr (Accessed October 30, 2011)

Chapter 9: Opiods, the Fear of Addiction and Treatment Agreements

41. M. Noble, et al., "Long-term opioid management for chronic noncancer pain," *Cochrane Database of Systematic Reviews* 1 (January 20, 2010):CD006605.

42. The National Opioid Use Guideline Group, *Canadian Guideline for Safe and Effective Use of Opioids for Chronic Non-Cancer Pain* (2010): 10.

43. *The American Society of Addiction Medicine*, "Definition of Addiction." http://www.asam.org/research-treatment/definition-of-addiction (Accessed November 13, 2012)

44. Karen Lee Richards, "Opioids: Addiction vs. Dependence." *HealthCentral.com*, http://www.healthcentral.com/chronic-pain/coping-279488-5.html (Accessed October 2, 2010)

45. Ibid.

46. Christopher D. Prater, Robert G. Zylstra, and Karl E. Miller, "Successful Pain Management for the Recovering Addicted Patient," *The Primary Care Companion to the Journal of Clinical Psychiatry* 4, no. 4 (2002): 125–131. http://www.ncbi.nlm.nih.gov/pmc/articles/PMC315480/ (Accessed October 2, 2010)

47. Thank you to Toronto Police 51 Division for clarifying this issue.

48. Megan Ottman, "Migraines, Pain, and Narcotics Contracts: What to Do if You're Terminated." *HealthCentral.com*, http://www.healthcentral.com/migraine/doctors-511054-5.html (Accessed October 16, 2010)

49. *International Association For the Study of Pain*, "Declaration That Access to Pain Management Is a Fundamental Human Right." http://www.iasp-pain.org/Content/NavigationMenu/Advocacy/DeclarationofMontr 233al/default.htm (Accessed October 1, 2011)

Chapter 11: Side Effects from Top to Bottom

50. Yvonne Nestoriuc, E. John Orav, Matthew H. Liang, Robert Horne, and Arthur J. Barsky. "Prediction of nonspecific side effects in rheumatoid arthritis patients by beliefs about medicines," *Arthritis Care & Research* 62, no. 6 (February 26, 2010): 791–799.

Chapter 13: Mood Swings and Mental Gymnastics

51. Carol Eustice, "Does Prednisone Tapering Minimize Withdrawal?" *About.com: Rheumatoid Arthritis*, http://arthritis.about.com/od/prednisone/f/withdrawaltaper.htm (Accessed June 23, 2011)

52. Eric Reynolds, "Three Breath Relaxation Technique." *Mindbody Pain Clinics*, http://mindbodypainclinics.com/three-breath-relaxation-technique/ (Accessed July 3, 2011)

Chapter 14: Sinuses

53. Seth Schwartz, "Sinusitis." *MedlinePlus*, http://www.nlm.nih.gov/medlineplus/ency/article/000647.htm (Accessed July 7, 2011)

54. Odessa Gill, N.D, personal communication.

Chapter 15: Asthma and Allergies

55. Leslie Alderman, "Who Should Worry About Dust Mites (and Who Shouldn't)." *New York Times*, http://www.nytimes.com/2011/03/05/health/05patient.html (Accessed March 31, 2012)

Chapter 16: Hypertension, Strokes and Heart Attacks

56. Claire Bombardier, et al. for the VIGOR Study Group, "Comparison of Upper Gastrointestinal Toxicity of Rofecoxib and Naproxen in Patients with Rheumatoid Arthritis," *The New England Journal of Medicine* 343, no. 21 (2000): 1520–1528, 2 p following 1528.

57. *Heart and Stroke Foundation*, "Stroke Warning Signs." http://www.heartandstroke.com/site/c.ikIQLcMWJtE/b.3483937/k.772A/Stroke__Warning_Signs.htm (Accessed July 12, 2010)

58. *Heart and Stroke Foundation*, "Heart Attack Warning Signals."
     http://www.heartandstroke.com/site/c.ikIQLcMWJtE/b.3483917/k.
     171E/Heart_disease__Heart_Attack_Warning_Signals.htm,
     (Accessed July 12, 2010)

Chapter 17: Managing Infection Risk

59. Alexandra, "I Finally Got the Point... My Summer Vacation..."
     HealthCentral.com, http://www.healthcentral.com/rheumatoid-
     arthritis/c/234279/85345/vac (Accessed July 1, 2010)

60. *The Johns Hopkins Lupus Center*, "Things To Avoid."
     http://www.hopkinslupus.org/lupus-info/lifestyle-additional-
     information/avoid/ (Accessed September 23, 2012)

61. *Wheels.ca*, "Gas Pump Handles Top Study of Filthy Surfaces."
     http://www.wheels.ca/columns/article/800800 (Accessed
     November 13, 2011)

Chapter 18: Nausea and Acid

62. Sharon Gillson, "Proton Pump Inhibitors (PPIs)." *About.com*,
     http://heartburn.about.com/od/medsremedies/a/protonpumpPPIs.
     htm (Accessed March 21, 2012)

63. *University of Rochester Medical Center*, "Ginger Quells Cancer
     Patients' Nausea From Chemotherapy."
     http://www.urmc.rochester.edu/news/story/index.cfm?id=2491
     (Accessed September 23, 2012)

Chapter 19: Gas

64. *Beano*, "Beano FAQs."http://www.beanogas.com/en/about-
     beano/beano-faqs.aspx (Accessed September 23, 2012)

65. *Gas-X*, "Gas-X Frequently Asked Questions (FAQs)."
     http://www.gas-x.com/faqs.jsp (Accessed December 12, 2012)

Chapter 21: Dryness, Thirst and Skin Care

66. *The Arthritis Society,* "Sjögren's Syndrome." http://www.arthritis.ca/page.aspx?pid=1002 (Accessed September 23, 2012)

67. *WebMD,* "Dental Health and Dry Mouth." http://www.webmd.com/oral-health/guide/dental-health-dry-mouth (Accessed May 5, 2012)

68. *MedicineNet.com,* "Definition of Lichenification." http://www.medterms.com/script/main/art.asp?articlekey=10131 (Accessed July 9, 2011)

Chapter 22: Bladder

69. Katrina Woznicki, "Cranberry Juice Fights Urinary Tract Infections Quickly." *Web MD,* http://women.webmd.com/news/20100823/cranberry-juice-fights-urinary-tract-infection-quickly (Accessed May 27, 2012)

70. *WebMD,* "Bladder Spasms." http://www.webmd.com/urinary-incontinence-oab/bladder-spasms (Accessed July 9, 011)

Chapter 23: Hormones, Sex Drive and Other Unmentionables

71. Lisa Emrich, "RA and Sex: Could Estrogen Levels or Methotrexate Affect Your Sex Life?" *HealthCentral.com,* http://www.healthcentral.com/rheumatoid-arthritis/c/72218/112875/life (Accessed July 25, 2010)

72. Ibid.

73. Ibid.

74. D. Gordon, G.H. Beastall, J.A. Thomson, and R.D. Sturrock, "Prolonged Hypogonadism in Male Patients with Rheumatoid Arthritis during Flares in Disease Activity," *British Journal of Rheumatology* 27, no. 6 (December 1988):440–444.

75. Robert L. Brent, "Teratogen Update: Reproductive Risks of Leflunomide (AravaTM); A Pyrimidine Synthesis Inhibitor: Counseling Women Taking Leflunomide Before or During Pregnancy and Men Taking Leflunomide Who Are Contemplating Fathering a Child," *Teratology* 63 (2001): 106–112.

Chapter 24: Weight Changes

76. *What Health*, "How to Calculate BMI." http://www.whathealth.com/bmi/formula.html (Accessed July 4, 2011)

77. Ibid.

78. Lene Andersen, "The Arthritis Foundation: Changing the Future of Arthritis." *HealthCentral.com*, http://www.healthcentral.com/rheumatoid-arthritis/c/80106/137764/fou (Accessed July 4, 2011)

Chapter 25: Osteoporosis

79. Coburn Hobar and Jessica B. Johnson, "Hormone Replacement and Osteoporosis." *Emedicinehealth*, http://www.emedicinehealth.com/hormone_replacement_and_osteoporosis/article_em.htm (Accessed July 20, 2010)

80. Miranda Hitti, "Acid Reflux Drugs May Up Fractures." *WebMD*, http://www.webmd.com/heartburn-gerd/news/20080811/lengthy-use-of-reflux-drugs-may-up-fractures (Accessed June 24, 2012)

81. *Canada's Food Guide*, "How Much Food You Need Every Day."
    http://www.hc-sc.gc.ca/fn-an/food-guide-aliment/basics-
    base/quantit-eng.php (Accessed July 20, 2010)

82. *National Institutes of Health Office of Dietary Supplements*,
    "Calcium." http://ods.od.nih.gov/factsheets/Calcium-
    HealthProfessional/ (Accessed June 24, 2012)

83. Ibid.

84. *EatRight Ontario*, "Calcium Supplements."
    http://www.eatrightontario.ca/en/Articles/Bone-Health/Calcium-
    Supplements.aspx (Accessed June 24, 2012)

85. Ibid.

86. *National Institutes of Health Office of Dietary Supplements*,
    "Calcium." http://ods.od.nih.gov/factsheets/Calcium-
    HealthProfessional/ (Accessed June 24, 2012)

87. *National Institutes of Health Office of Dietary Supplements*,
    "Vitamin D." http://ods.od.nih.gov/factsheets/vitamind-
    HealthProfessional/ (Accessed June 11, 2012)

88. Lene Andersen, "Rheumatoid Arthritis and Osteoporosis:
    Preventing and Managing Thinning Bones. " *HealthCentral.com*,
    http://www.healthcentral.com/rheumatoid-
    arthritis/c/80106/116877/ra (Accessed July 4, 2011)

89. Pam Flores, "Osteoporosis Medications." *HealthCentral.com*,
    http://www.healthcentral.com/osteoporosis/c/76444/123832/osteo
    porosis (Accessed June 24, 2012)

Chapter 26: A Hodgepodge of Other Side Effects

90. Carol Eustice, "Can Hair Loss Caused by Arthritis Medications Be
    Prevented or Treated?" *About.com*,
    http://arthritis.about.com/od/arthritismedications/f/hair_loss.htm
    (Accessed June 10, 2012)

91. Timothy Gower, "Methotrexate: Managing Side Effects." *Arthritis Today*, http://www.arthritistoday.org/conditions/rheumatoid-arthritis/ra-treatment/methotrexate-side-effects.php (Accessed June 19, 2012)

92. Carol Eustice, "What Causes and Heals Mouth Sores in Arthritis Patients?" *About.com*, http://arthritis.about.com/od/arthritissignssymptoms/f/mouthsores.htm (Accessed June 19, 2012)

93. Timothy Gower, "Methotrexate: Managing Side Effects." *Arthritis Today*, http://www.arthritistoday.org/conditions/rheumatoid-arthritis/ra-treatment/methotrexate-side-effects.php (Accessed June 19, 2012)

94. *Mayo Clinic*, "Shingles." http://www.mayoclinic.com/health/shingles/DS00098 (Accessed June 21, 2012)

95. European League Against Rheumatism, "Treatment with Anti-TNFs Can Increase the Risk of Shingles by up to 75%." *Science Newsline*, http://www.sciencenewsline.com/articles/2012060714410016.html (Accessed June 21, 2012)

96. Liam Davenport, "Rheumatism drugs may increase shingles risk." *News Medical*, http://www.news-medical.net/news/20120615/Rheumatism-drugs-may-increase-shingles-risk.aspx (Accessed June 21, 2012)

97. *Centers for Disease Control and Prevention*, "Shingles Vaccine: What You Need to Know." http://www.cdc.gov/vaccines/vpd-vac/shingles/vacc-need-know.htm (Accessed June 21, 2012)

98. *Mayo Clinic*, "Shingles." http://www.mayoclinic.com/health/shingles/DS00098 (Accessed June 21, 2012)

99. Ibid.

Chapter 27: Rare and Serious Side Effects

100. Allison Tsai, "Q&A: Pregnancy and Rheumatoid Arthritis." *HealthCentral.com*, http://www.healthcentral.com/rheumatoid-arthritis/c/888425/112033/qp (Accessed July 5, 2012)

101. P.R. Crook, "Leflunomide Therapy," *gp-training.net*, http://www.gp-training.net/rheum/therapy/leflun.htm (Accessed July 27, 2010)

102. Robert L. Brent, "Teratogen Update: Reproductive Risks of Leflunomide (AravaTM); A Pyrimidine Synthesis Inhibitor: Counseling Women Taking Leflunomide Before or During Pregnancy and Men Taking Leflunomide Who Are Contemplating Fathering a Child," *Teratology* 63 (2001): 106–112.

103. Tammy Worth, "Studies Show Anti-TNF Drugs Don't Raise Cancer Risk." *Arthritis Today*, http://www.arthritistoday.org/news/anti-tnf-cancer-risk142.php (Accessed July 6, 2012)

104. Ibid.

105. Andrea Kane, "FDA Adds New Anti-TNF Infection Warnings." *Arthritis Today*, http://www.arthritistoday.org/news/anti-tnfs-warning154.php (Accessed July 7, 2012)

106. Jordan Lite, "What is Histoplasmosis?" *Scientific American*, http://www.scientificamerican.com/article.cfm?id=what-are-fungal-infection (Accessed July 9, 2011)

107. Ibid.

108. *National Institute of Diabetes and Digestive And Kidney Diseases,* "Cirrhosis." http://digestive.niddk.nih.gov/ddiseases/pubs/cirrhosis/ (Accessed July 7, 2012)

109. *FDA*, "FDA Drug Safety Communication: New boxed warning for severe liver injury with arthritis drug Arava (leflunomide)." http://www.fda.gov/Drugs/DrugSafety/PostmarketDrugSafetyInfor mationforPatientsandProviders/ucm218679.htm (Accessed July 9, 2011)

110. *Centers for Disease Control and Prevention*, "Drug-Resistant TB." http://www.cdc.gov/tb/topic/drtb/default.htm (Accessed July 7, 2012)

Chapter 31: Pain Management Specialists

111. Jan Carstoniu, "Chronic Pain and Multidisciplinary Treatment." *HealthCentral.com*, http://www.healthcentral.com/rheumatoid-arthritis/c/401444/105385/mu (Accessed December 27, 2010)

112. Jan Carstoniu, "About Doctors (#5-Using Doctors)." *Mindbody Pain Clinics*, http://mindbodypainclinics.com/using-doctors-series/about-doctors-5-using-doctors/ (Accessed December 27, 2010)

Chapter 33: Acupuncture

113. *Acupuncture Foundation of Canada Institute*, "Welcome to AFCI." http://www.afcinstitute.com/ (Accessed July 17, 2011)

Chapter 34: Massage and Touch

114. Cathy Wong, "Massage Therapy." *About.com Alternative Medicine*, http://altmedicine.about.com/od/treatmentsmtoq/a/massage.htm (Accessed July 17, 2011)

115. Steven D. Ehrlich, "Massage." *University of Maryland Medical Center*, http://www.umm.edu/altmed/articles/massage-000354.htm (Accessed January 2, 2011

116. *Massage.ca*, "FAQ: Frequently Asked Questions About Massage Therapy." http://www.massage.ca/f_a_q_.html (Accessed January 2, 2011)

117. *Massage.ca*, "Contraindications and Cautions for Massage Therapy Treatment." http://www.massage.ca/contraindictionscautions.html (Accessed January 2, 2011)

118. *American Massage Therapy Association*, "Starting a Career in Massage Therapy: What You Need to Know." http://www.amtamassage.org/professional_development/starting.html (Accessed July 16, 2011)

119. Crystal Hawk, "Therapeutic Touch: A Healing Lifestyle." *Therapeutic Touch*, http://www.therapeutictouch.com/tt1.html (Accessed January 2, 2011)

120. *The International Center for Reiki Training*, "What is Reiki?" http://www.reiki.org/FAQ/WhatIsReiki.html (Accessed July 17, 2011)

Chapter 35: Meditation

121. *The Transcendental Meditation Program*, "Maharishi Mahesh Yogi." http://www.tm.org/maharishi (Accessed July 17, 2011)

122. *MailOnline*, "Meditation 'Reduces the Emotional Impact of Pain Making It Easier to Bear.'" http://www.dailymail.co.uk/health/article-1283445/Meditation-reduces-emotional-impact-pain-making-easier-bear.html (Accessed January 8, 2011)

123. Jon Kabat-Zinn, *Mindfulness for Beginners* (Sounds True, Incorporated Unabridged Audiobook, 2006)

124. Thanks to Dr. Jan Carstoniu for this brilliant description of meditation.

Chapter 36: Managing Your Energy

125. Christine Miserandino, "The Spoon Theory." *But You Don't Look Sick*, http://www.butyoudontlooksick.com/articles/written-by-christine/the-spoon-theory/ (Accessed November 4, 2011)

126. *Johns Hopkins*, "Rheumatoid Arthritis." http://www.johnshopkinshealthalerts.com/symptoms_remedies/rheumatoid_arthritis/94-1.html (Accessed September 3, 2012)

Chapter 37: Filters, Focus and Fun

127. Mark McGuinness, "Why Multitasking Doesn't Work." *Lateral Action*, http://lateralaction.com/articles/multitasking/ (Accessed March 5, 2011)

Chapter 38: Surgery

128. *American College of Rheumatology*, "People with Rheumatoid Arthritis Have Less Joint Surgery Compared to 25 Years Ago." http://www.rheumatology.org/about/newsroom/2009/2009_am_16.asp (Accessed March 13, 2011)

129. *WebMD*, "Arthroscopy for Rheumatoid Arthritis.," http://www.webmd.com/rheumatoid-arthritis/arthroscopy-for-rheumatoid-arthritis#aa18752 (Accessed October 7, 2012)

130. *WebMD*, "Synovectomy for Rheumatoid Arthritis." http://www.webmd.com/rheumatoid-arthritis/synovectomy-for-rheumatoid-arthritis (Accessed March 13, 2011)

131. Lisa Emrich, "Soft-Tissue Surgery in Rheumatoid Arthritis: Synovectomy, Tendon Repair, and Carpal Tunnel Release." *HealthCentral.com*, http://www.healthcentral.com/rheumatoid-arthritis/c/72218/130129/soft (Accessed October 12, 2012)

132. Ibid.

133. William C. Shiel, Jr., "Carpal Tunnel Syndrome and Tarsal Tunnel Syndrome." *MedicineNet.com*, http://www.medicinenet.com/carpal_tunnel_syndrome/article.htm (Accessed October 7, 2012)

134. Lisa Emrich, "Soft-Tissue Surgery in Rheumatoid Arthritis: Synovectomy, Tendon Repair, and Carpal Tunnel Release." *HealthCentral.com*, http://www.healthcentral.com/rheumatoid-arthritis/c/72218/130129/soft (Accessed March 13, 2011)

135. *WebMD*, "Joint Fusion Surgery (Arthrodesis) to Treat Arthritis." http://www.webmd.com/osteoarthritis/guide/joint-fusion-surgery (Accessed October 7, 2012)

136. Lisa Emrich, "What Types of Surgery Are Used in Rheumatoid Arthritis?" *HealthCentral.com*, http://www.healthcentral.com/rheumatoid-arthritis/c/72218/128668/rhe (Accessed March 13, 2011)

Chapter 39: Physical Therapy

137. *Canadian Physiotherapy Association*, "What We Do." http://thesehands.ca/index.php/site/What_Do_Physiotherapists_Do/ (Accessed March 19, 2011) Note: The text on this website has since been changed, but this exact definition of physical therapy appears on numerous websites explaining the discipline. It was not possible to find the original source.

138. Lene Andersen, "Keeping Mobile: Physical Therapy & RA." *HealthCentral.com*, http://www.healthcentral.com/rheumatoid-arthritis/c/80106/132585/ra (March 19, 2011)

139. Lene Andersen, "Keeping Mobile: Physical Therapy & RA," *HealthCentral.com*, http://www.healthcentral.com/rheumatoid-arthritis/c/80106/132585/ra (Accessed March 19, 2011)

Chapter 40: Occupational Therapy

140. *The American Occupational Therapy Association, Inc.*, "About Occupational Therapy." http://www.aota.org/Consumers.aspx (Accessed March 28, 2011)

141. Dena Slonaker, "A More Comfortable Splint." *Arthritis Today*, http://www.arthritistoday.org/community/expert-q--a/rheumatoid-arthritis/more-comfortable-splint.php (Accessed October 18, 2012)

142. Byrd McDaniel, "What Are Hand Splints?" *eHow Health*, http://www.ehow.com/about_4795233_hand-splints.html (Accessed November 3, 2012)

143. *The American Occupational Therapy Association, Inc.*, "Ergonomics." http://www.aota.org/Consumers/consumers/Work/Ergonomics.aspx (Accessed March 28, 2011)

Chapter 42: Living Your Life with RA

144. Thank you to Leslie Vandever for this brilliant analogy.

145. Dickinson, Emily, *Hope*.

Your Life with Rheumatoid Arthritis

Your Life with Rheumatoid Arthritis